D0573771

# MEDITATION
## • MADE SIMPLE •

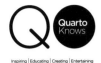

Brimming with creative inspiration, how-to projects, and useful information to enrich your everyday life, Quarto Knows is a favorite destination for those pursuing their interests and passions. Visit our site and dig deeper with our books into your area of interest: Quarto Creates, Quarto Cooks, Quarto Homes, Quarto Lives, Quarto Drives, Quarto Explores, Quarto Gifts, or Quarto Kids.

This edition published in 2019 by Crestline,
an imprint of The Quarto Group
142 West 36th Street, 4th Floor
New York, NY 10018 USA
T (212) 779-4972 F (212) 779-6058
www.QuartoKnows.com

First published in 2016 by Fair Winds Press, an imprint of The Quarto Group,
100 Cummings Center, Suite 265-D, Beverly, MA 01915, USA.

10 9 8 7 6 5 4 3 2 1

ISBN: 978-0-7858-3776-3

Digital edition published in 2016

eISBN: 978-1-63159-209-6

Design: Mattie Wells

Printed in China

# MEDITATION
## · MADE SIMPLE ·

Weekly Practices for Relieving Stress,
Finding Balance, and Cultivating Joy

PAULA WATKINS, Ph.D.

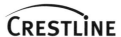
CRESTLINE

# Contents

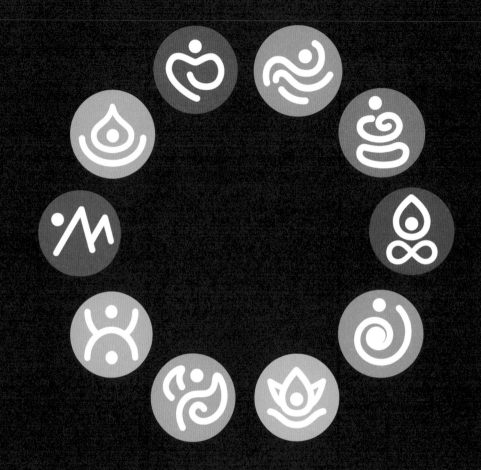

# INTRODUCTION

SINCE YOU'VE PICKED UP THIS BOOK, IT'S LIKELY THAT YOU'VE ALREADY HEARD ABOUT THE MANY BENEFITS OF MEDITATION: MANAGING STRESS, CULTIVATING A SHARPER MIND, OR ENHANCING YOUR QUALITIES OF EMPATHY AND COMPASSION. NOT ONLY IS MEDITATION AN EASY AND EFFECTIVE WAY TO HELP US MEET THE DEMANDS OF OUR FAST-PACED LIFESTYLES, BUT IT CAN ALSO HELP US BE THE BEST VERSION OF OURSELVES. IT CAN OPTIMIZE HOW WE ARE, WHO WE ARE, AND WHAT WE OFFER TO EACH OTHER AND TO THE WORLD. AND IT MAY SURPRISE YOU TO LEARN THAT VAST RESERVOIRS OF PEACE AND PRESENCE EXIST WITHIN EACH OF US—NO MATTER HOW CHAOTIC THINGS MAY SEEM ON THE SURFACE OF OUR LIVES.

The practices in this book will help you rediscover these inner resources. You'll be guided through fifty-two different meditation and mindfulness practices—and you'll be encouraged to experience, experiment with, and explore meditation for yourself, in the ways that work best for you.

## WHAT IS MEDITATION?

Meditation is mind training and the term refers to a group of practices that all share a key feature: They're intended to cultivate the mind in some way, such as to promote relaxation, encourage mental clarity, and expand to one's sense of vibrancy, awareness, and connectedness.

# PATHWAYS TO MEDITATION

First of all, there's more than one way to meditate. *The Vijnana Bhairava Tantra*—one of the most ancient and key texts on meditation in the Kashmir Shaivism tradition—is a great example of the many forms meditation takes: It contains 112 different meditation techniques, including breath awareness, chanting, visualization, and contemplation. And different cultures around the world have developed their own practices for training the mind through meditation. These include the Buddhist, Hindu, and yoga paths (which are often thought of as a single entity, but which are, in fact, unique) as well as the Jewish Kabbalah, Christian, and Sufi traditions, plus myriad Indigenous systems, which include various Aboriginal, Native American, and African communities. While the specifics of these traditions vary, all meditation practices worldwide train the mind in ways that help quiet the noise of normal daily mental activity. Essentially, meditation trains our minds to become more stable, subtle, and supple so that we can experience different aspects of our consciousness.

People often raise their eyebrows at the word *consciousness*, but it simply means "awareness," and meditation changes the quality or state of our awareness. Here's how that happens. We can describe our normal day-to-day level of awareness as "gross" or "rough." At this level, the more delicate aspects of our experience are generally overlooked because our mind is in "doing mode," absorbed in all of the to-do lists, targets, chores, plans, and activities that clamor for our attention. It's perfectly normal (and necessary) for our minds to focus on such material aspects of day-to-day life, but it can also get pretty exhausting. Minds can quickly become saturated, overstimulated, and overworked. It's also easy for them to feel disconnected from the bodies that host them, from the other people around them, and from the great world in which they live. Our gross level of awareness is also incredibly time bound and falls prey to the modern fear of time famine: the fear that time is going too fast, and that we can't and won't get everything done. (Sound familiar?) While we all know that there's little to be gained from fearing time, it's still a modern-day epidemic, and it leaves us feeling stressed, depressed, anxious, and irritated.

Thankfully, meditation can help. It allows us to re-immerse ourselves in "deep time" and enter into "being mode," rather than "doing mode." It refines our awareness so that we become conscious of the subtler aspects of life. Meditation invites us to let go of our chronic overidentification with the surface aspects of our lives as the sums of our identity. It frees us from being ruled by our own minds, and from an idea of self that's composed only of "I," "me," and "mine." It enables us to disengage from the mental chatter that constantly flows through our minds and to experience infinitely more expansive aspects of our life and existence.

In meditation, we simply come to "be." We're not striving to be better than another person—or even better than ourselves. We rest our busy, analytical minds; in doing so, we become present to the deeper rhythm and pulse of life that is always available to us when we turn inward. What's more, scientific studies have shown that meditation promotes good physical health, sharper mental and cognitive functioning, emotional and psychological well-being, and healthy relationships and behavior.

## MEDITATION AND MINDFULNESS: WHAT DO THEY MEAN?

There's an ongoing debate among scholars regarding the uses and meanings of the terms *meditation* and *mindfulness*. It's a tricky situation, because both have multiple definitions, and they inevitably overlap. (The debate even extends into issues of translation from Pali and Sanskrit texts into English!) While we don't need to enter into the scholarly specifics of this debate, it's still important to understand the history of these terms and how they're being used in contemporary Western settings.

The term *meditation* generally refers to the practice of formally setting time aside to cultivate or train the mind, and there are countless ways to do so. For example, you might choose to focus your mind on your body, your breath, a mantra, or a prayer. One of the best-known types of meditation is called "mindfulness," which means paying attention to the present moment with an open, nonjudgmental attitude. Mindfulness has been adapted from its traditional Buddhist context and has been promoted for several decades by Western psychologists and medical professionals as a way to enhance physical and mental health.

Mindfulness can be practiced in two ways: formally, in classical seated meditation, or informally, by bringing greater awareness to your day-to-day activities. Informal mindfulness practices focus on how we apply the openness, presence, and nonreactivity cultivated during formal meditation practice to the rest of our lives. In this sense, meditation and mindfulness both overlap and complement one another, since they could be viewed as two different facets of the same concept. Scholars will continue to debate this issue for years to come, but in my view—and for the purposes of this book—the term *mindfulness* reminds us that meditation isn't just something that happens when our eyes are closed. It's a dynamic practice that can and should be used in everyday life, and that's why you'll find both formal and informal meditation and mindfulness practices throughout this book.

## HOW TO USE THIS BOOK

This book takes an eclectic approach to meditation, drawing on techniques and teachings from a variety of spiritual traditions. This, I hope, will encourage you to explore the vast world of meditation, to discover your personal preferences, and to tune in to the similarities and differences between approaches. According to some schools of thought, a mixture of techniques is discouraged and students are advised to stick with a single tradition and a single teacher, but I believe that it's up to each individual to discover what resonates with her or him.

That's why *Meditation Made Simple* offers a wide sample of approaches; it's meant to act as a starting point for anyone who's interested in knowing more about training the mind and opening the heart through meditation. It doesn't assume that you have any prior knowledge or experience, so it's structured in a way that will make meditation easy and effective. These fifty-two practices follow a progression—from introductory to intermediate levels—and you can journey through the book over the course of a year by immersing yourself in one practice per week, or you can approach each chapter as an individual unit. Feel free to choose any chapter or practice that appeals to you at any time. You may find that you spend 3 days on certain practices and 2 weeks on others. That's fine. The weekly structure isn't arbitrary. Meditation is a personal journey. Here's a quick rundown of what you'll find:

- In chapter 1, you'll become familiar with breath awareness, the cornerstone of meditation.

- Chapter 2 will introduce you to the concept of mindfulness and help you become grounded—that is, fully present—in your own body.

- In chapter 3, you'll learn to stabilize your mind during meditation with the use of an anchor, which can help you focus your awareness.

- Chapter 4 shows you how to witness, or become aware, of your own thoughts and their impact on your experience.

- Chapter 5 is all about open awareness, and asks you to remain present to your own experience as you meditate. (Don't worry; it's not as hard as it sounds!)

- In chapter 6, you'll find that meditation isn't always about sitting still. Moving meditations are a great way to bring mindfulness and intention to your daily activities.

- Chapter 7 will help you rethink your relationship with physical pain and to manage it more successfully with meditation.

- Chapter 8 guides you toward a more thoughtful, less habitual, way of dealing with difficult emotions—the sticky, tricky ones you'd rather avoid.

- Chapter 9's focus is equanimity—the art of staying balanced and composed, no matter what's going on around you.

- In chapter 10, you'll become familiar with the concept of loving kindness, which is central to most spiritual traditions, and you'll learn to embrace it in your daily practice.

Each of these chapters contains three elements: the formal meditation practices themselves; the informal Mindful Living Tips that'll help you integrate the skills you've learned into your everyday life; and the Key Concept sections that will support your practice and deepen your understanding of meditation. You'll also find Spotlight on Science notes interspersed throughout the book. These quick excerpts from recent scientific research into meditation and its benefits are there to boost your motivation and provide a little extra inspiration. Then, at the end of the book, there's a Q&A section that addresses some common questions and concerns about meditation.

## MATERIALS AND TIPS

You already have everything you need for meditation: a mind and body. Honestly, you don't need anything else but the following tips and guidelines will help you get off to the best start.

### LET GO OF "PERFECT"

As you work your way through the meditations in this book, try to remember that there's no such thing as perfection—and that's as true for your meditation practice as it is for your daily life. So, don't feel that you need to complete all of these practices perfectly or to the letter of the instructions. Relax: Read them, try them, and follow the spirit of them in the way that works best for you.

## POSTURE

When it comes to meditation posture, the most important rule is to be comfortable—but not so much so that you feel like falling asleep. It's all about balance; you want to be comfortable and relaxed, yet wakeful and alert.

- Sit in an upright position and, unless necessary, don't let your back or neck lean against anything. If necessary, you can provide some support for your lower back, like a cushion, bolster, or blanket. Try not to lie down, since you'll be more likely to fall asleep that way.

- It's best to raise your hips slightly, by sitting on a cushion or bolster.

- Relax your shoulders, rest your hands on your lap or thighs, and balance your head evenly. If you're feeling drowsy, try lifting your chin a little; if your mind is racing, lower your chin slightly.

- Don't punish yourself with an unpleasant posture that simply doesn't work for your body.

- The last—and best—tip for good posture is this: Hold an inner smile behind your lips and eyes. You don't have to smile with your whole mouth; just imagine the smile to yourself, and lift the corners of your mouth a bit. Doing this will help you stay positive and focused throughout your practice.

## GENERAL COMFORT

- Avoid meditating on a full stomach or after taking stimulants such as caffeine or sugar.

- Have a blanket nearby if you're likely to get cold.

- Make sure that your clothing is not constrictive—loose is best.

- Find some solitude and limit disturbances as much as possible. Turn off your phone or set it on silent, and close the door to the room you're in.

## WHEN AND WHERE

In terms of *when*, the answer is anytime, really. Morning practices are great—they set us up with an optimal physiology and mind state to start the day, and they're typically harder to avoid as the distractions and demands of our day have yet to begin. Late at night is probably the trickiest, as we can be prone to falling asleep. Many meditators find that first thing in the morning and/or early evening tend to be achievable rhythms. Others shut the office door or walk to the park during their lunch hour. The most important thing is to find a time that works for you and, ideally, establish a routine, as we are creatures of habit after all.

As for the question of *where* to practice, I suggest setting yourself up for success by finding a quiet environment where you are unlikely to be disturbed. While complete silence is not a requirement for meditation in the beginning, quieter environments are certainly easier.

## HOW TO BEGIN

Always begin each meditation practice by taking some time to settle your body and deepen your breath. Some gentle stretches or yoga postures can help prepare the body, and in chapter 1 you'll master a series of breathing practices that you can use to prepare your body and mind for meditation.

## HOW TO USE THE INSTRUCTIONS AND GUIDELINES

Read through the instructions for each practice to get an idea of what's required, but once you begin your meditation don't obsess about the specifics. Reread only if you really need to. Instead, focus on the spirit of the practice. (If you're trying a practice for the first time, you might like to record the instructions on your smartphone and play them back to yourself.)

## HOW TO END

At the end of your meditation practice, sit with your eyes closed in silence for a few moments. Let go of the object or concept of your meditation. Become aware of your body and your surroundings. You might wish to reflect on how you feel after your practice. Whatever your experience, try not to judge or attempt to change it. Just notice the effect of your meditation practice on your internal state. Gently begin to move or stretch your body, slowly open your eyes, then mindfully rise up to transition back into your activities.

Meditation can be life changing. Let's begin!

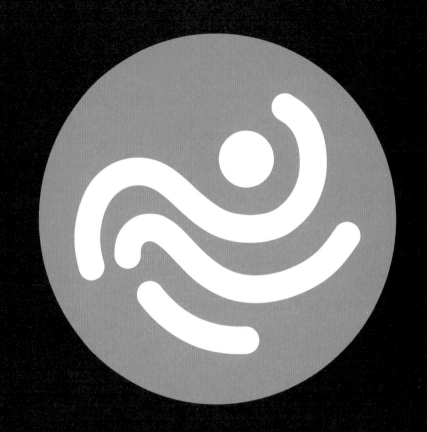

:: CHAPTER 1 ::

# CALLING CALM

BREATH AWARENESS IS CENTRAL TO MOST MEDITATION TECHNIQUES. IN SOME TRADITIONS, THE BREATH BECOMES THE CENTRAL OBJECT OF FOCUS FOR THE MEDITATION, AND IN OTHERS, BREATH AWARENESS IS SIMPLY USED AT THE BEGINNING OF PRACTICE TO BECOME GROUNDED AND CENTERED BEFORE ENTERING INTO MEDITATION. EITHER WAY, BREATHING IS A VITAL ASPECT OF MEDITATION, WHICH IS WHY THIS CHAPTER IS DEVOTED ENTIRELY TO DEVELOPING BREATH AWARENESS.

Breathing is more crucial to life than eating or drinking. We can survive for weeks without food and for days without water, but only for a few minutes without breath. Surprisingly, though, it isn't something we generally think or talk much about—perhaps because it happens so naturally and instinctively, and because it requires no conscious effort. However, because the act of breathing sits directly at the interface between our **voluntary** and **autonomic nervous systems**, it's a powerful way for us to use our bodies to communicate very quickly with our brains. Breathing is where body and mind intersect, and it's also something we can consciously and easily manipulate. We can speed it up, hold it, or slow it down, and when we do these things, we experience direct physical, mental, and emotional effects.

The **autonomic nervous system** oversees bodily functions over which we don't have conscious awareness or control, such as digestion and temperature regulation. The **voluntary nervous system**, on the other hand, relates to aspects of our physiology that are under our conscious control, such as using our muscles to move our arms and legs.

The importance of breathing correctly has long been overlooked by Western science, but most other health traditions have always emphasized it. In India, for example, within **Ayurvedic** medicine and yoga traditions, the art and science of consciously manipulating the breath is a key practice. It's known as

**pranayama**, which means "extension of breath" or "extension of the life force." Ancient Sanskrit texts from India offer some of the most detailed analyses of breath work practices. Many of these practices are only now being explored and understood by the Western scientific community, and the research to date demonstrates that they do enhance physical, mental, and emotional well-being. (We'll explore some of that research—and the practices themselves—later on in this chapter.)

---

**Ayurveda** is India's traditional system of medicine and healing.

---

*Ayur* = life

*Veda* = science/knowledge

**Pranayama** is a type of yogic breath awareness and regulation. It is a Sanskrit term meaning "extension or channeling of life force."

*Prana* = vital life force

*Yama* = to control/to practice self-control

## CALM BREATHING

The calm breathing exercises in this chapter will teach you to activate your **parasympathetic nervous system**—the wing of the greater autonomic nervous system with the important job of promoting rest, repair, and relaxation throughout the body. When the parasympathetic nervous system is activated, your overall oxygen consumption, heart rate, and blood pressure all decrease. One way to activate your parasymphathetic nervous system is through deep breathing: Long, slow, even

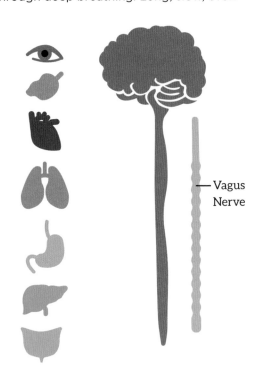

Vagus Nerve

**Parasympathetic Nervous System**

exhalations stimulate the **vagus nerve** (*vagus* means "wandering" in Latin), which literally wanders from the brainstem all the way down through the neck and into the abdomen. (While the vagus nerve is usually referred to in the singular, there's actually one nerve on each side of the body.) It connects nearly every major organ, including the tongue, heart, lungs, and intestines, and, when it's stimulated by a big, full, and complete exhalation, it triggers the release of cortisol and endorphins in the brain and generally helps you chill out.

This combination of an alert but relaxed mind, brain, and body takes us into the experience of flow, primes us for peak performance in all of our daily tasks, and, quite simply, prepares us to be the best and most beautiful we can be. It's also a powerful tool for calling both mind and body into meditation.

## ❶ KEY CONCEPT: PATIENCE

Patience is an attitude that can really help you with mindfulness and meditation, and it's also a skill you'll develop as you practice. Patience reflects an understanding and acceptance that things must unfold in their own time—although, in this era of efficiency, fast food, and instant communication, it's hardly a quality that Western culture promotes!

In this chapter, you'll begin to explore this key concept and attitude by practicing patience toward your breath. That might sound pretty easy—and in some ways, it is. You'll be

encouraged to watch your breath and follow each inhalation and exhalation to its natural conclusion, and for some people, this might seem to take a painfully long time. That familiar feeling is called impatience, and it will arise in both body and mind as you practice, but that's okay. If you're new to meditation, you might find this hard to believe, but the truth is, cultivating patience doesn't mean rejecting impatience. In fact, observing impatience is a useful way to develop and strengthen patience.

---

**Patience:** the ability to calmly accept and tolerate delay or difficulty.

---

What does impatience look like? It can manifest as a feeling of irritation, agitation, disappointment, and frustration. You might also notice it as a thought that pops into your mind, such as "This is taking too long!" or, "When will this finish?" Keep an eye out for thoughts like these as you watch your breath, and let them ebb and flow. Try to accept that both your breath and your sense of impatience will unfold in their own time. Being mindful of impatience in this way doesn't eradicate it, but it does help us respond to it skillfully when it occurs. The presence of impatience invites us to choose to act in a way that's more consistent with bringing greater calm, clarity, presence, and patience into our lives.

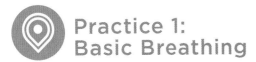

# Practice 1: Basic Breathing

This basic breathing technique is officially known as **diaphragmatic breathing**, but you can think of it simply as a "calming breath." It's the most common method psychologists use to effectively treat stress, anxiety, and insomnia. Many people find that it becomes their go-to technique for lowering stress levels and preparing mind and body for meditation.

## TECHNIQUE

1.  This technique can be practiced while sitting, lying on your back, or even while standing. Your eyes may be either open or closed, whichever feels right to you.

2.  Take a moment to loosen and soften your body, especially the shoulders, upper chest, and jaws. Bring your awareness to each of these parts of the body. Then relax any tenseness or tightness you find there. Imagine your breath softening any knots or tight areas.

3.  Bring your awareness to your breath, and focus on breathing in through the nose and out through the mouth.

4.  Now, begin to lengthen your breath to a 6-second cycle: that is, breathe in for 3 seconds and out for 3 seconds.

5.  Rest one hand on your belly and the other on your chest.*

**Diaphragmatic breathing**—also known as abdominal, belly, or deep breathing—promotes respiratory effectiveness. It's accomplished by contracting and expanding the diaphragm, a muscle located between the chest cavity and the stomach cavity. During this type of breathing, the belly expands as air enters the lungs.

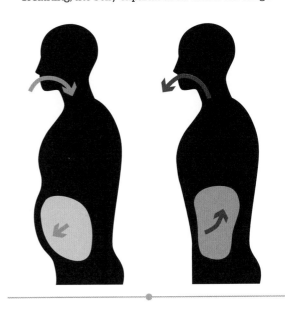

*ALTERNATIVELY, PLACE BOTH HANDS ON EITHER SIDE OF THE UPPER RIB CAGE WITH THE FINGERS APPROXIMATELY 1 INCH (2.5 CM) APART. AS YOU INHALE, NOTICE THAT THE HANDS EXPAND SIDEWAYS AS THE LUNGS FILL AND AS THE RIB CAGE EXPANDS BOTH FORWARD AND SIDEWAYS. AS YOU EXHALE, NOTICE HOW YOUR FINGERTIPS MOVE CLOSER TOGETHER AGAIN.*

6. As you inhale through your nose, let your waist and stomach expand outward. The hand on the abdomen should rise. In contrast, the hand on your chest should hardly move at all.

7. As you exhale slowly through your mouth, the abdomen should move downward, or flatten, as it naturally contracts. In contrast, the hand on your chest should hardly move at all.

*This completes one round. Repeat steps 4 through 7 as many times as you wish. When you are finished, relax both arms and breathe*

---

**Kumbhaka** is a Sanskrit term that refers to the yogic pranayama practice of breath retention or intentionally holding the breath.

---

*naturally for a few moments before opening your eyes, if you've closed them.*

## INTERMEDIATE OPTIONS

When you're confident with the basics of relaxed breathing, you can begin to change the timing of your breath, introduce pauses or holds (known as **kumbhaka** in yoga), and learn to isolate and activate different muscles within the torso.

As you explore these intermediate techniques, always be sure to prioritize smooth, even breathing.

### SPOTLIGHT ON SCIENCE

Every part of your body needs oxygen to survive, but that's especially true for your brain. Although the brain comprises only about 2 percent of your total body weight, it receives 15 to 20 percent of your blood supply. So, by breathing fully, completely, and correctly, you'll promote optimum blood oxygenation, which, in turn, contributes to a well-fed, fully awake brain.

### TIMING

Aim to increase (and eventually double) the length of your exhalation in comparison to your inhalation. For example, IN: 2 and OUT: 4 or IN: 3 and OUT: 6.

### PAUSING

Introduce gentle pauses at the end of the inhalation and at the end of the exhalation. For example, IN: 4, HOLD: 2, OUT: 6, HOLD: 2

###  PRACTICE TIPS

Aim to practice this technique for 3 to 5 minutes at least once, but preferably twice, per day.

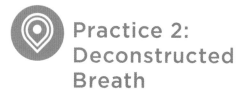

## Practice 2: Deconstructed Breath

This practice encourages you to explore the lower, middle, and upper regions of the torso through your breath. The aim is to breathe sequentially into each area, filling the lower torso first and then gradually allowing the breath to fill the entire rib cage and chest area. Each exhalation follows this pattern in reverse, deflating from the top areas first and emptying the lower torso last.

### TECHNIQUE

1. Sit or kneel comfortably. Your eyes may be open or closed, whichever feels right to you.

2. Soften your body, especially the shoulders, upper chest, and jaws. Bring your awareness to each of these parts of the body in turn. Then loosen, soften, and relax any tenseness or tightness you find there.

3. Begin to breathe in and out through your nose.

4. As you inhale, draw about one-third of the breath into your lower belly. Allow your waist and stomach to expand outward. Draw another one-third of the inhalation into your rib cage, allowing the ribs to expand to the front, sides, and back of the torso. Draw the last one-third of your inhalation into your upper chest, allowing your sternum to rise slightly.

5. On your exhalation, release one-third of the breath from your upper chest first. Notice that your sternum sinks down slightly. Release another one-third of the breath from the rib cage and allow the rib cage to recede toward the center of your body. Release the final one-third of your exhalation from your lower belly.

*This completes one round. Repeat the pattern of steps 4 and 5 as many times as you wish. When you are finished, simply sit still and breathe naturally for a few moments before opening your eyes, if you've closed them.*

### ⬡ PRACTICE TIPS

Aim to practice this technique for 3 to 5 minutes at least once, but preferably twice, per day.

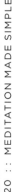

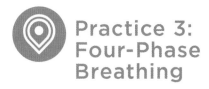

## Practice 3: Four-Phase Breathing

We typically think of the breath cycle in terms of inhalations and exhalations, but the truth is, every breath is also composed of natural "holds" or turning points—small but significant pauses in which the breath shifts from inhalation *to* exhalation and exhalation *to* inhalation. The practice of four-phase breathing is an invitation to explore these natural turning points in the breath, and it is offered here with the traditional Sanskrit terms for each of the four stages.

### TECHNIQUE

1. Sit or kneel comfortably with your eyes open or closed, whichever feels right to you.

2. Soften your body as in Practice 2, and begin breathing in and out through the nose.

3. **Phase 1: Inhalation (*puraka*).** Inhale smoothly. Imagine that you're drinking the air as if it were water. Follow the inhalation to its completion.

4. **Phase 2: Pause after inhaling (*abhyantara kumbhaka*).** Pause at the top of the inhalation, holding the air in the lungs and exploring the sense of fullness and completeness that arises in this moment.

5. **Phase 3: Exhalation (*rechaka*).** Exhale smoothly, effortlessly relaxing all of the muscles in your torso.

6. **Phase 4: Pause after exhaling (*bahya kumbhaka*).** Pause intentionally at the end of the exhalation. Before you begin a new cycle of breathing, explore this empty moment and the way in which it is full of potential.

*This completes one round. Repeat the pattern from steps 3 to 6 as many times as you wish. When you are finished, simply sit still and breathe naturally for a few moments before opening your eyes, if you've closed them.*

*You may experience some discomfort during the first few times you try this technique, particularly if you pause for too long in steps 4 and 6 and then feel the need to rush to complete the next inhalation or exhalation. This suggests you're holding each pause for too long. With practice, you'll soon be able to remain calm and relaxed throughout the practice.*

### ⚫ PRACTICE TIPS

Aim to practice this technique for 3 to 5 minutes at least once, but preferably twice, per day.

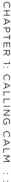

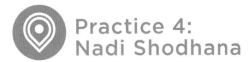

## Practice 4: Nadi Shodhana

The technique of *Nadi Shodhana*, often called "alternate nostril breathing," has a venerable history in Ayurvedic medicine and yoga. It's thought to bring the two hemispheres of the brain into harmony with one another, resulting in balanced physical, mental, and emotional well-being. Modern science has yet to adequately understand this practice, but what's clear is that nostril dominance affects brain activity and that *Nadi Shodhana* has positive effects on cardiovascular and pulmonary health.

We all experience natural fluctuations in nostril airflow during the course of each day, with the right or left nostril being more dominant at different times. This widely studied phenomenon is known as the nasal cycle, and *Nadi Shodhana* effectively manipulates this naturally occurring pattern in order to stimulate and change the nervous system.

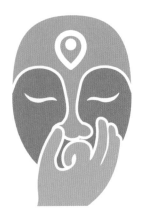
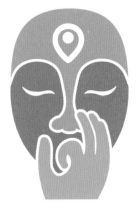

### TECHNIQUE

1.  Sit in any position that's comfortable for you. Relax the body and breathe naturally for a few moments, allowing your mind and body to settle.

2.  Rest your left hand on your lap or knee.

3.  Make a "peace sign" with your right hand. Place your right thumb gently onto your right nostril. Place your right ring and little fingers gently onto your left nostril. Fold the two extended fingers toward the palm or rest them lightly on the bridge of your nose.

4.  Close your eyes and begin by softly closing your right nostril with your right thumb. Inhale slowly, deeply, smoothly, gently, and without strain through your left nostril.

5.  Close your left nostril using your right ring and little fingers, and release your right nostril. Exhale through your right nostril.

**Nadi Shodhana,** or "alternate nostril breathing," is a scientifically researched breathing practice that brings balance to mind and body.

**6.** Inhale through your right nostril. Close your right nostril and release your left. Exhale through your left nostril.

*This completes one round. Repeat the pattern from steps 4 to 6 at least twice. When you are finished, simply sit still and breathe naturally for a few moments before opening your eyes.*

## INTERMEDIATE OPTIONS

When you are confident with the basics of alternate nostril breathing, you can begin to explore these variations.

### TIMING

Aim to increase (and eventually double) the length of your exhalation in comparison to your inhalation. For example: IN: 2 and OUT: 4 or IN: 3 and OUT: 6.

### PAUSING

Introduce gentle pauses at the end of the inhalation and at the end of the exhalation. For example: IN: 4, HOLD: 2, OUT: 4, HOLD: 2.

### SPOTLIGHT ON SCIENCE

Scientists began exploring *Nadi Shodhana* in the 1980s and 1990s, and found that nostril dominance is associated with greater electrical activity in contralateral brain hemispheres, with improved performance on cognitive tasks and with emotional tones reflecting the function of the hemisphere in question.

## ⬤ PRACTICE TIPS

Aim to practice this technique for 3 to 5 minutes at least once, but preferably twice, per day. Your first practice can be done in bed right after you wake up in the morning, and your second practice can also take place in bed, when you're about to rest for the night. Alternatively, you might like to set an alarm or reminder on your smartphone to help you remember to practice throughout the day.

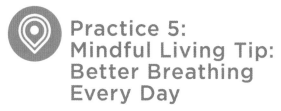

## Practice 5: Mindful Living Tip: Better Breathing Every Day

Whether you practice meditation formally or not, spending a few minutes each day on breathing exercises is a wise investment of your time. And calm breathing principles can be used throughout the day, too. Here's how to integrate calm breathing into your everyday activities.

### SET REMINDERS

Set up to five reminders to yourself throughout your day, encouraging you to "just breathe" for around 60 to 90 seconds. This practice helps you learn to tune in to your body, to relax on cue, and to develop the habit of infusing your daily activities with greater calm.

There are several great apps for creating smartphone reminders: download your favorite one, and use it. Or write reminders to yourself on Post-It notes and stick them on your desk, in your bathroom, or beside the kettle to remind yourself to soften your belly, drop your shoulders, and breathe long, low, and slow down into the abdomen.

### USE AS NEEDED

Use these techniques as needed wherever and whenever you could benefit from turning the

stress dial down to low. For instance, if you find yourself in the middle of a challenging meeting, you could gently relax your belly and begin to lengthen and slow your breath. Alternatively, you could take a bathroom break and give yourself a moment to get grounded by implementing your calm breathing techniques.

### THE CALMER COMMUTE

The time we spend getting to and from work provides us with the perfect opportunity to practice breathing techniques. You can easily do them in public, too; your fellow commuters won't even notice. Just keep your eyes open as you focus on lengthening, deepening, and softening each breath.

### DRESS FOR SUCCESS

Some styles of clothing can make it difficult to relax your abdomen for optimal breathing. Never fear: that doesn't mean that you have to wear your baggiest sweaters and loosest pants to work every day! Just remember to loosen your belt or pop open the top button on your pants or skirt when you're sitting at your desk. That way, you'll be able to breathe deeply and fully, so your brain and body can function at their peak.

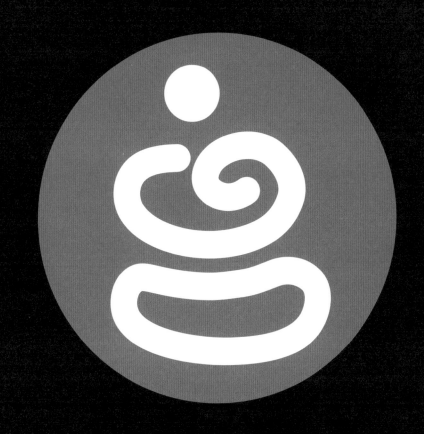

:: CHAPTER 2 ::
# GETTING GROUNDED

NOW THAT YOU'VE TUNED INTO THE PRESENCE OF YOUR BREATH, IT'S TIME TO TURN YOUR ATTENTION TO THE CONCEPT AND PRACTICE OF MINDFULNESS. IN THIS CHAPTER, YOU'LL LEARN MINDFUL BODY AWARENESS TECHNIQUES TO GET YOU GROUNDED IN THE PRESENT MOMENT. YOU'LL ALSO BEGIN TO AWAKEN YOUR SENSES IN ORDER TO FULLY EXPERIENCE THE RICHNESS OF THE WORLD AROUND YOU.

There are many ways to practice mindfulness, and you'll experience dozens of them throughout this book. The foundational and traditional mindfulness practices offered here in chapter 2 are designed to help stabilize your mind and provide you with a foundation for further meditation training. Through practicing these techniques, many people discover that there's so much more beauty and wonder in their daily lives than they ever thought possible (at least, as an adult!). That's because the human mind tends to become a little lazy—habituated to, and even unimpressed with, the array of wonders available to our senses on a daily basis. Meditation can help you break out of that rut and rekindle your love affair with life.

That's where the practices in this chapter come in. They're intended to be "grounding"—that is, they bring us into the reality of the present moment through inviting us back into our bodies. Our body is our home and our vehicle, and it is the medium through which we experience and interact with this life. And yet we often tend to live inside our heads,

barely aware of what we're experiencing at the physical level. Sometimes, we nearly forget that we *have* bodies at all—and we lose sight of the fact that our bodies are mirrors for the state of our emotional and psychological well-being.

## ❶ KEY CONCEPT: MINDFULNESS

Mindfulness is actually a very simple concept: it is a way of paying attention. When we practice mindfulness meditation, we use a nonjudgmental attitude to pay attention, on purpose, to the present moment.

The *"on purpose"* part of this statement tells us that mindfulness involves **consciously** directing our awareness, by actively deciding where and what to focus on. That's the very opposite of being lost in a wandering mind or stuck on automatic pilot.

The *"present moment"* part tells us that we pay attention to the here and now. It also clues us in to the fact that our minds could be somewhere else—a feeling we're all familiar with. Our minds can be in the future, in the past, or right here and now, experiencing life as it unfolds. In mindfulness, we're concerned with noticing what's going on right now.

Finally, the **"nonjudgmental"** aspect lets us know that being mindful means we make no attempt to evaluate experiences or to classify them into good, bad, right, or wrong, and this can be a challenge. It can also be a great and valuable lesson, because key sources of our distress lie in our unwillingness to accept life as it is and in our desire to control all of our experiences.

While the majority of mindfulness practices utilized in the Western world today have their roots in Buddhist traditions, being mindful isn't an explicitly Buddhist practice, and you don't need to adhere to a specific belief or tradition in order to do it. In fact, being mindful isn't even exclusive to meditators. Being mindful is a basic human ability and experience. The human mind has an inherent capacity to pay attention to the present moment, so mindfulness practices simply enhance our already present ability to be mindful. Within Western science, mindfulness meditation is the meditation technique that has attracted the most research. It has been formally integrated into Western health care since the late 1970s, and research continues to demonstrate that it can enhance physical and mental health and well-being.

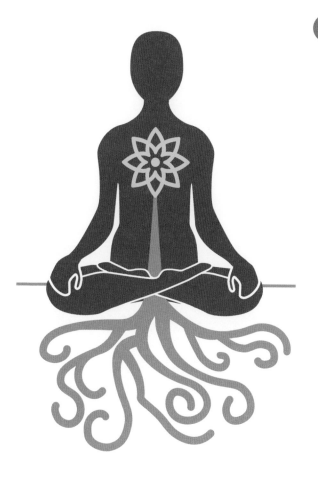

To be **grounded** means to be fully present in your body and your current experience in the now.

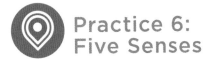

# Practice 6:
# Five Senses

The five senses practice will help you feel grounded, come to your senses (literally!) and be in the present moment. It offers a gentle inroad into a relaxed but alert mind state—the foundational mind state of meditation. Through it, you'll also begin practicing the fundamental attitudes of mindfulness by cultivating your capacity to bring spaciousness, freedom, and curiosity to whatever you experience.

## TECHNIQUE

1. Sit in any position that's comfortable for you.

2. Enjoy three full, conscious breaths, and then let your breathing settle into a natural rhythm. Try not to force your breath: simply allow the breath to breathe itself.

3. Now bring your attention to everything you hear. Notice the sounds around you. First, take note of the loudest, or most prominent, sound you can detect. Then begin to observe all of the quieter sounds in your immediate environment. Pay attention to the faintest sound you can detect. This might even be a sound that's located within your own body. Notice the sounds around you with an attitude of nonjudgmental openness and curiosity. Become interested in the sheer sensory discovery.

4. Then, shift your attention and focus all of your awareness on everything you can smell. Bring the same attitude of nonjudgmental openness and curiosity to your awareness. Again, begin by noticing the most prominent smell you can detect. (It's okay if you can't detect any particular scent right now; just notice this experience as the absence of smell and accept this as your experience in the present moment.) Explore your sense of smell, but do so without analysis. Maybe there's a fragrant rose garden right outside your window, or maybe a friendly family of skunks has taken up residence in your backyard. Either way, try not to label the smells you notice as "good" or "bad." Simply be wide open to what you are experiencing.

5. Move your attention and awareness to everything you can taste. Try to explore this sense with a wide-open attitude of curiosity toward your experience, just as you did with your senses of hearing and smell. You might not notice any particular taste as you're doing this: if so, that's fine. Allow that to be your experience. You're practicing awareness without analysis by simply noticing what you notice.

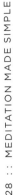

6. Now, shift your attention and focus all of your awareness on your sense of touch. Bring your awareness into your body and curiously notice what you notice. Explore prominent sensations (perhaps aches or pains), and then take your awareness on a body-wide journey. Investigate the subtle sensations within your body and on your skin. Maybe you feel the itch of a mosquito bite on your right arm, or you sense that your left foot might be about to fall asleep. Or perhaps you feel your stomach gurgling. Whatever it is, notice it with a welcoming attitude of nonjudgmental openness and curiosity.

7. Lastly, shift your attention to your sense of vision. Begin to explore everything you can perceive. (You can still keep your eyes closed if you wish; simply begin to notice with curiosity everything you see behind the eyelids.) If you can't see anything, accept that, too. Either way, explore your sense of vision, but without analysis. Be wide open to whatever you experience.

8. When you're ready to complete your practice, relax your awareness for a few moments before opening your eyes.

## ⬤ PRACTICE TIPS

Formal Practice: Practice daily for 10 to 20 minutes, spending 2 to 4 minutes exploring each sense.

Informal Practice: Once you're familiar with the practice, you'll be able to use five senses throughout your day. For example, as you're walking to work, shift your attention to the sights, smells, tastes, tactile sensations, and sounds around you, spending from 30 seconds to 3 minutes on each sense.

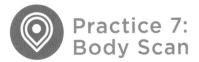

# Practice 7: Body Scan

The body scan is a foundational mindfulness meditation practice in which you'll learn to purposefully guide your attention to notice different parts of your body. It is not a relaxation practice (although relaxation is often one of its by-products). Instead, its aim is to encourage you to be curious about your experience and simply take note of any sensations you observe—without judging the experience or attempting to change it.

As you move through the body scan, try to be simply there with whatever's happening. Just notice whatever you notice. For example, feel the moisture behind your eyelids and on your tongue; notice the warmth of that light sunburn on the back of your neck; pay attention to the gentle rumbling in your belly. This may sound simple, but it can be harder than it seems. That's because we often respond to our bodies by judging our physical sensations—especially if we encounter pain or discomfort—and then we try to change the experience or distract ourselves from fully encountering it. But with practice, we can become fully aware of, and curious about, whatever's going on in our bodies. Try to be openhearted and accepting of the sensations you discover during the body scan, no matter how comfortable or uncomfortable they might be. (For a handy list of some of the sensations that might arise during body scan practice, see the table on page 32.)

## TECHNIQUE

1. Sit or lie down in any position that's comfortable for you.

2. Take a few moments to soften your body by loosening and relaxing any tension or tightness you sense. Breathe consciously for a few moments, allowing your mind and body to settle. Feel the contact your body is making with the floor or chair.

3. Now bring your attention to your head. Feel the weight of your head on your neck, and pay attention to the physical sensations surrounding it. Notice any sensation at all: heat, cold, itching, pain, tightness, tension, looseness, or even tickling. Observe all of these sensations without judging them as good, bad, right, or wrong. Then shift your awareness from your head as a whole and

begin to explore the head area part by part. Start with the crown of your head, then move to the forehead, the eyes, temples, nose, cheeks, and mouth. Explore the inside of the mouth and the chin. If you feel your mind racing, don't worry: simply acknowledge it, and gently draw your attention back to a specific part of your body.

4. Move your attention to your neck. First, explore the sensations in the entire neck area, and then, part by part, travel to the front, sides, and back of the neck. Notice the sensations on the surface of the skin on your neck, as well as those that lie deeper within the throat.

5. Now turn your attention to your shoulders and explore the entire shoulder area. Then let your awareness move part by part into your left arm, elbow, wrist, hand, and fingers. Repeat on the right arm. Try to stay aware of your moment-to-moment experience, noticing all the sensations that arise with an attitude of curiosity, and remember that it's perfectly normal for your mind to wander. When you become aware that your mind has wandered, just gently guide it back to the part of the body you were exploring.

6. Next, bring your awareness to your torso. Begin with the chest area and notice the subtle movement of your chest as you breathe. Explore the front, back, and sides of your rib cage. Notice the pressure of your back against the floor or chair. As you move down your torso, your awareness might pick up on any

sensations in the abdomen and stomach, from the deep interior to the surface.

7. Shift your attention to the lower back and pelvis, the hip bones, genitals, and groin. Again, without judgment, simply notice whatever sensations arise.

8. Continue to direct your attention downward, and become aware of your buttocks. Feel them press against the chair or floor. Bring your awareness to your left thigh, and feel

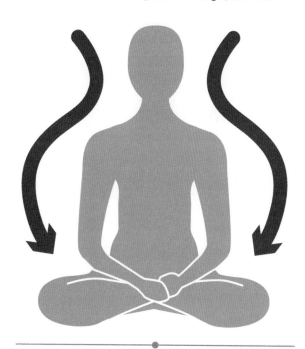

The body scan practice helps to bring your awareness into the present moment.

its weight and strength. Notice any other sensations as you continue to shift your attention down to your knee, shin, calf, ankle, foot, and toes. Repeat on the right leg.

9. Now it's time to widen your focus and turn your attention toward your body as a whole. As you inhale, fill your whole body with breath and awareness, and begin to sweep your attention from your feet to your head and back again. Extend your awareness and experience to your entire body.

## ○ PRACTICE TIPS

Formal Practice: Practice daily for 10 to 20 minutes. Depending on the time you have available for this exercise, spend 1 to 3 minutes on each major region of the body (that is, your head, neck/throat, left arm and hand, right arm and hand, torso, pelvis, left leg and foot, and right leg and foot).

Informal Practice: Once you're familiar with this practice, you'll be able to enjoy a quick and grounding body scan any time of day. Move through your body, part by part, or simply tune in to the body as a whole and notice the sensations that present themselves.

What kinds of sensations arise during the body scan practice? This table might help you cultivate mindful awareness of the different sensations you may encounter.

| PHYSICAL SENSATIONS YOU MIGHT ENCOUNTER | | | | |
|---|---|---|---|---|
| Achy | Dense | Light | Shaky | Tender |
| Bruised | Dull | Loose | Shivery | Tense |
| Bubbly | Dry | Nauseous | Stinging | Tight |
| Burning | Fluttery | Numb | Soft | Tingling |
| Buzzing | Hot | Prickly | Sore | Trembling |
| Cool | Heavy | Pounding | Spacey | Throbbing |
| Cold | Itchy | Pulling | Spacious | Twitchy |
| Clammy | Icy | Pulsing | Sweaty | Uncomfortable |

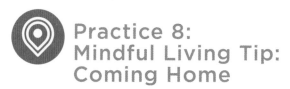

# Practice 8:
# Mindful Living Tip:
# Coming Home

Throughout this chapter, you've been cultivating your ability to call your awareness home and into the present moment, as it is within your body during formal meditation practice. Here are some extra tips to help you practice coming home to the body—and the present moment—in everyday life.

## THE CONSCIOUS COMMUTE

Whether you walk or ride during your daily commute, take yourself on a journey through each of your five senses (see page 28) as you move toward your office or workplace. Since it's typically the easiest one to begin with, start with your sense of vision. For instance, noticing orange and yellow autumn leaves falling from the trees as you walk. Noticing these leaves might bring up childhood memories of school—but try not to lose yourself in those memories. Instead, draw your attention back to your senses—to the crisp scent of autumn in the air, or the way the breeze feels on your nose and cheeks.

## SEATED SCAN

You can perform a seated scan just about any time you find yourself sitting down: in the car (keep your eyes open if you're driving!), at your desk, or on a train. Depending on how much time you have, you can move through your body part by part, as you did in Practice 7, or you can sweep over your body from feet to head and back again, simply noticing sensations and letting them go.

Although this isn't strictly a mindful body scan technique, you can add a little muscle relaxation as you move your awareness throughout your body. Release, loosen, and soften any tense areas you come across. (You might be surprised at how much unnecessary tension you carry in your shoulders, neck, and jaw during the course of daily life!)

## BEDTIME BLISS

The practices in chapter 2 are lovely rituals to help you settle your awareness into your body before sleep. Try one or both, and bring your day to a close by returning your awareness to your body—away from the busy realm of doing, planning, and organizing.

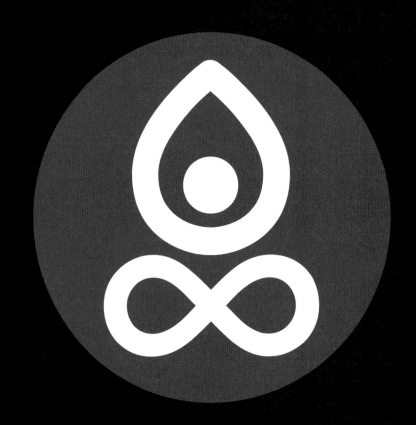

:: CHAPTER 3 ::

# ANCHORING
# AWARENESS

YOU'VE LEARNED HOW TO DRAW YOUR ATTENTION BACK TO THE PRESENT MOMENT. NOW YOU'LL EXPLORE CLASSICAL MINDFULNESS AND MEDITATION TECHNIQUES THAT STABILIZE AND SETTLE THE MIND AND ANCHOR YOUR AWARENESS. THESE PRACTICES ARE TAUGHT AS THE FIRST STAGES OF MEDITATION IN BUDDHIST AND YOGA TRADITIONS, WHERE THEY'RE KNOWN AS *SAMATHA* AND *DHYANA*, RESPECTIVELY. THE PRACTICES IN THIS CHAPTER WILL PROVIDE YOU WITH A FOCUS OR ANCHOR ON WHICH YOU CAN REST YOUR ATTENTION AS YOU BEGIN THE JOURNEY OF OBSERVING AND SETTLING YOUR MIND.

## BENEFITS OF ANCHORING AWARENESS

The benefits of these meditation practices can be grouped into four key areas: physical health; mental and cognitive functioning; emotional and psychological well-being; and interpersonal and social relationships. Let's take a closer look at each.

**Samatha** is the Buddhist term for the practice of calming the mind through focusing on a single object. **Dhyana** is one of the eight limbs of classical yoga. It, too, refers to the practice and state in which the mind is steadied by the use of some sort of object of contemplation.

## PHYSICAL HEALTH

- Deep relaxation and activation of the parasympathetic nervous system, which leads to lowered heart rate, blood pressure, and respiration

- Enhanced immune functioning and accelerated rates of healing

- Decreased pain

- Slowed cellular effects of aging and stress through enhanced cell longevity

## MENTAL AND COGNITIVE FUNCTIONING

- Increased focus

- Decreased distractibility

- Enhanced memory

- Improved fine-motor coordination

- Greater creativity

## EMOTIONAL AND PSYCHOLOGICAL WELL-BEING

- Enhanced self-awareness

- Increased emotional self-regulation

- Less distress from negative, unhelpful, and overly analytical thoughts

- Greater positive emotionality: gratitude, love, and compassion

- Reduced relapse rates and improved well-being in the treatment of patients with a range of conditions, including depression and anxiety

## INTERPERSONAL AND SOCIAL RELATIONSHIPS

- Stronger self-awareness in relationships

- Enhanced perspective taking (that is, the ability to understand, appreciate, and empathize with a number of different perspectives that may not be identical to your own)

- Greater social responsiveness

- Enhanced empathy

- Increased compassionate behavior

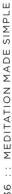

## ⓘ KEY CONCEPT: EFFORTLESS EFFORT

The idea of effortless effort might seem like a paradox. The concept of effortless effort asks us to set aside our usual achievement-oriented way of approaching our activities. It invites us to give up the need to control, and it teaches us to refrain from forcing any kind of experience that isn't naturally happening during meditation. As we do this, we allow the meditation to unfold and happen by itself. All we need to do is provide the right conditions and let the mind's gravitational pull toward deeper stillness take over.

The nature of the mind is such that it becomes quieter when we create the right conditions for it to do so, just as a muddy pond will become clear when the conditions are right. If we keep stirring the pond, the mud will continue to float and cloud the surface. However, if we simply allow the floating particles of dirt to drift and dance, they'll eventually make their way to the bottom of the pond to rest in stillness. We must apply both patience and effortless effort as we allow the mud to settle; if we try to *force* it to settle and be still, we'll just end up creating more chaos. Similarly, if we dive into the mind and attempt to chase away thoughts or command them to be quiet, we'll simply stir up further mental noise. If we sit back and allow thoughts to come and go as they please, over time we create the conditions in which the mind can begin to settle and to experience moments of stillness.

Effortless effort isn't synonymous with laziness. Instead, it's an embodiment of the recognition that forceful striving isn't always the best approach. True, you might be instructed to "focus" or even "concentrate" your mind during meditation—but the fact is, these English-language terms are very limited translations for the type of awareness you're being called to employ. The true purpose of meditation isn't to cultivate a mind that's particularly brilliant at merely concentrating on one thing. Being able to steady your awareness is simply one aspect of meditation. Whenever you come across the words *focus* or *concentrate* in relation to meditation, remember also the concept of effortless effort, and find a middle path between the two.

Here are some more tips to help you create the ideal conditions for "effortless effort" in meditation:

- **Effortless effort doesn't mean that you should stop yourself from thinking**, or even that you need to make yourself more relaxed. Meditation really becomes an effortful struggle only when people believe that their thoughts need to be cleared away. The truth is that meditation has nothing to do with obliterating the mind's ability to think. We come to enter the great peace of meditation by learning how to be an observer of the thinking mind.

- **Use a meditation anchor**—you'll learn how later on in this chapter—and focus on it softly and faintly, but diligently. Use a light touch and rest your awareness on your meditation anchor gently. Do not attempt to grasp the anchor forcefully: there's no need to concentrate on it in the traditional sense of the word. Simply rest your awareness on it. and never focus on your meditation anchor in an attempt to stop your thoughts.

- **Take a few moments to settle down and breathe** before beginning your meditation. Revisit the techniques in chapter 1, if you like.

- **Let go of any expectations or preferences** you might have about your meditation practice. Take each moment as it comes. Remember, when it comes to meditation—and life in general—there's no such thing as perfect.

- **Be physically comfortable** (see the introduction) and adjust your posture throughout your meditation, if necessary.

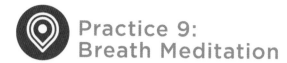 ## Practice 9: Breath Meditation

### THE BREATH AS ANCHOR

The breath is a popular object for meditation for several sensible and beautiful reasons. First of all, the breath is your life partner. It's with you during every moment of your life, including the most challenging ones. You don't need to seek it out—it's already there. All you need to do is turn your attention toward it. It is always in the present moment, and you can connect to it silently. No one around you needs to notice what you're doing.

---

Your breath sits at the intersection of your body and your mind. It reflects the state of your nervous system and sensitively responds to changes in your physical and emotional experience. You can gain a better understanding of your emotional landscape through attunement to the breath.

---

Secondly, our breath is a gauge for our nervous system. It reflects the shifts and changes within our bodies and minds on a moment-to-moment basis. When we're anxious, it speeds up. In moments of ecstasy, it hangs suspended at the end of the inhalation. When we're deeply rested, it can soften to a barely detectable flutter. A mindful connection to the breath can help you tune in to the state of your nervous system in all life situations—and, if necessary, it can allow you to shift your emotional and mental state to one of greater clarity and calm.

Thirdly, breath requires no belief system. You don't have to accept anything about it or its powers. You just have to pay attention to it—and it's already happening, during each and every second of your life. Another good reason for focusing on very faint aspects of the breath, such as the breath around the nostrils, is that the delicate nature of the experience prepares you for further meditation practices that require an increasingly refined and subtle awareness of your senses and your physical being.

## THE MIRACLE OF RESPIRATION

Breathing might seem like a pretty boring activity to most people, most of the time—but it's actually quite an astounding thing, since every breath involves the interaction and communication of trillions of cells. In the womb, our lungs were filled with fluid, and we obtained oxygen through our bellies via our umbilical cords. But within seconds after birth, we gasped as our central nervous systems first came into contact with this new way of breathing and being. We inhaled, and our lungs inflated all on their own, moving oxygen into our bloodstream and removing carbon dioxide from it with exhalation. This beautiful, intricate dance will continue without any conscious effort on our parts for every moment of our lives. Our lives begin with an inhalation and will end with an exhalation. The breath, literally, breathes us.

Without breath, there is no life. Breath is life pulsing within us—but do we really experience it fully? All meditation traditions instruct practitioners to bring awareness to the act of breathing (in fact, one of my teachers poetically guides students to "*drink* the breath"). When we experience the essence of life moving inside us, it becomes clear that every moment and every breath is a precious, if not miraculous, phenomenon. From this perspective, then, the apparently ordinary act of breathing is truly an extraordinary process.

It's all too easy for these important messages to sound cliché—but they're repeated so often for a reason. Becoming a dance partner with the breath is truly one of the quickest, easiest, and most time-tested (as well as scientifically validated) ways to enter into meditation. And when we enter into this dance, we must remember that the breath is the leading partner. We merely follow its rhythm. We don't try to change, dominate, or manipulate the breath during the practice of Breath Meditation. We simply turn up. That's how we become witnesses to this extraordinary pulsation of life within us as we cultivate the capacity to stabilize and settle our awareness.

## TECHNIQUE

1. Sit in any position that's comfortable for you and close your eyes.

2. As you become aware of the fact that you're breathing, draw your awareness to your breath.

3. Enjoy three full, slow, deep breaths. Fill the abdomen as you inhale, and allow your entire body to soften as you exhale. Then allow your breath to settle into a natural rhythm. There is no need to alter your breath; just observe it as it happens. Let the breath breathe you.

4. Notice the natural movement of your breath through the rise and fall of your abdomen and chest or through the subtle sensations of the breath around the nostrils. Choose one of these areas and rest your awareness there.

5. As you allow your awareness to rest on your breath, your mind will wander at some point—caught by distracting thoughts, external experiences, or bodily sensations. Perhaps you just remembered a task you forgot to finish before you left work, or maybe a fly has begun to buzz around the room, or you feel as if you're about to sneeze. That's perfectly normal. When you notice that this has happened, remind yourself that this experience is more than okay—in fact, it's an important part of the meditation process. Don't beat yourself up for letting your mind wander. Simply observe the distraction, and then gently bring your attention back to the breath. If you can do this, you're doing it right. Refrain from the urge to seek a completely still, settled mind. You might find it helpful to think of stillness as a stabilizing strength rather than a void in the mind's activity.

6. At the end of your practice, take a few moments to expand your awareness from the breath into the room around you. When you feel you're ready, open your eyes.

##  PRACTICE TIPS

Formal Practice: Practice daily for 10 to 20 minutes.

Informal Practice: Bring your full awareness to your breath at any moment throughout your day, and feel the centering power this timeless experience provides.

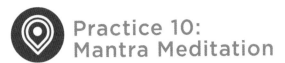 ## Practice 10:
## Mantra Meditation

If you've heard of mantra meditation before and feel a bit uneasy about it, set your worries aside. Consider this as an invitation to open your head and heart to a new perspective.

The meaning of the word *mantra* is "mind vehicle." In the Sanskrit language, *man* means "mind," while *tra* means "vehicle, tool, or instrument." Essentially, a mantra is a word or phrase repeated aloud or silently as an object of focus during meditation. Think of a mantra as a mechanism, an anchor, or an instrument that you can use as you transition from an excited, busy mind to a settled and restful, but alert, state of being.

## GOOD VIBRATIONS

According to the ancient yogic traditions of India, sound is the subtlest aspect of our experience as humans, and according to physics, those ancient traditions had it right. Before we go any further, here's a friendly warning: If you're concerned that we're about to launch into some version of the "universe as vibration" or the "all is one" cliché—well, strap yourself in! Remember, clichés develop for a reason. They're idioms that contain valuable kernels of truth.

Let's head back to the science for a moment. Quantum physics is based upon an understanding that any and all elementary particles possess a frequency or vibration. According to twentieth-century physicist Albert Einstein, everything in life is vibration, and since Einstein's time, scientists have studied atoms, quarks, leptons, and strings as they work toward a better understanding of our universe. We've since come to a point where molecular biologists—whose perspectives form the basis of our modern medical system—and physicists are in agreement with the ancient sages and modern mystics that the universe is, essentially, one grand symphony of sound.

## SOUND

Sound is a vibration that produces a wave of pressure through the air or through an object or medium, such as water. We're able to hear sound because this wave causes a very tiny vibration in our eardrums. Although we often refer to sound as the only waves of vibrations that can be heard by the human ear, it's true that our capacity to perceive sound is limited to a certain frequency, and that it differs to the capacity of other animals.

Music is a system of organized sound. We could also say that it's a system of organized vibration with a theoretical basis in arithmetic and geometry. What's more interesting to those of us who enjoy listening to it is how it affects us. We experience some vibrational frequencies as pleasant and the rest as "noise." We don't just "hear" music—we also "feel" it. It moves us both literally—when we dance to its beat—and emotionally. Certain frequencies of music, or organizations of vibrations, have been found to create a similar effect on listeners cross culturally. Generally, lower frequency sounds are experienced as more relaxing.

Significantly, throughout and across world religions, cultures, and languages, an interesting correlation arises between vowel sounds, meditative or prayer states, and parasympathetic nervous system activation. In Sanskrit, we have *aum*. In Islam, we find *amin* (pronounced ah-MEEN). Within Judeo-Christian traditions, we have *amen*. We also find universal sound expressions for our enjoyment of many sensory and sensual delights, from delicious food to sexual ecstasy.

## SACRED SOUND

Mantra meditation is typically associated with Indian religious thought (in the Vedic and Hindu traditions), but the use of sound to shift levels of awareness or consciousness likely predates these systems and may be traced to ancient Neolithic and, possibly, Paleolithic Shamanist traditions. Since the days of our ancient ancestors, we humans have believed in the sacred power of sounds and words as incantations, tools for altering mind states, and as a means for communicating with the divine.

Mantras might be "sound symbols" that represent a historical or an archetypal figure (known in Sanskrit as one's **Ishta devata**), or they may have no such association at all. When a mantra *is* associated with a person or deity, the meditator may visualize this figure as she chants the mantra, and in this way, the qualities associated with the figure are brought to mind. Many people find great benefit in cultivating a private and sacred relationship with a mantra and a spiritual figure in this way. For them, the mantra is like a seed planted in the soul. When the mantra is repeated, the seed is watered. In time, it grows into a great tree that can offer shelter during storms. With regular contemplation, the qualities of the deity may also become an increasingly common theme in the meditator's mind.

Mantras with a literal meaning—such as *shanti*, which translates as "peace"—may be chanted in the same way as those associated with a figure or deity, calling the qualities associated with the word or phrase to mind. In some traditions, mantras aren't used for their specific meaning—they may not even have a specific meaning—but are used instead for their sound or vibrational qualities. Vedic yogis are interested in using mathematics and astronomy to identify the vibration of the world at the time and place of a person's birth. They believe that this sound, when identified and used as a mantra, allows an individual to easily draw his or her attention inward and reconnect with a universal awareness that extends beyond space and time—that is, life or creation itself. This Vedic system, and other approaches to mantra meditation, are still practiced today in India and elsewhere in the world.

------

*Ishta devata* is a Sanskrit term denoting a worshipper's favorite deity. A mantra may be a word, sound, or phrase associated with a particular *Ishta devata*.

------

## TECHNIQUE

Before you begin, you'll need to choose a mantra to use. Some common mantras include *Aum, Aham* ("I am"), *Satya* ("truth"), and *So Hum* ("I am that," with "that" referring to all of creation). Alternatively, you could choose a word from any faith, such as *Amin, Shalom*, or *Amen*—or any word that has special beauty and meaning for you, such as *peace* or *surrender*.

1. Sit in any position that's comfortable for you and close your eyes.

2. Begin to recite your chosen mantra aloud.

3. Gradually turn down the volume on the mantra, but keep repeating it aloud. Then, turn down the volume so low that you're barely whispering. Now, turn down the volume until it's so faint and so fine that it's hardly more than an echo or gentle pulse in your mind. At this point, you are thinking the mantra.

4. As you allow the meditation to become softer and fainter, at some stage you'll forget about it altogether and begin thinking about something else. You may become distracted by thoughts or by noises in your environment—and that's completely normal. You're still practicing correctly: the drifting of the mind is actually an important part of meditation and shouldn't be resisted. When you realize that this has happened, simply return your attention to your mantra.

5. If you feel the mantra slipping away, that's okay. Just let it go, and then pick it up again.

6. At the end of your practice, keep your eyes closed for a few moments as you let go of the mantra. Expand your awareness to your breath, and then to the room around you. Open your eyes when you feel comfortable enough to do so.

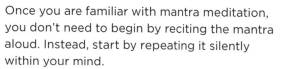

## ◍ PRACTICE TIP

Formal Practice: Practice daily for 10 to 20 minutes.

Once you are familiar with mantra meditation, you don't need to begin by reciting the mantra aloud. Instead, start by repeating it silently within your mind.

**"When the heart begins to recite, the tongue should stop."**

**—SUFI SAYING**

## Practice 11: Gazing Meditation

*Trataka*, meaning "to gaze," is another form of meditation that has its roots in India's yoga traditions. It involves anchoring the mind by focusing the gaze onto an external object, such as a candle. The idea behind this meditation is to develop a one-pointed focus (*dharana*), one of first the stages of meditation.

There are two phases to the practice of *trataka*. In the first, you'll focus your gaze on an object—in this example, we'll use a candle—until your eyes begin to water. In the second phase, you'll close your eyes and rest your attention on the afterimage of the candle in your mind's eye. Any external object may be used for *trataka*, including natural objects like the full Moon, a flower, or a stone. Objects of worship are also used for trataka and could include a picture of your chosen deity, or a **mandala** or **yantra**.

Some people find it easier to use a physical external anchor rather than the breath or a mantra, while others find open-eyed meditations like *trataka* a little bit tricky. Try it for yourself to see how you feel about this gazing meditation, and don't pressure yourself to continue if it doesn't feel right to you. (There are so many pathways for approaching meditation; you don't need to persist with a style that doesn't resonate with you.)

---

**Mandalas** and **yantras** are geometric patterns symbolically representing aspects of the universe or divinity, and are commonly found in Asian spiritual traditions. When using a mandala or yantra for *trataka* meditation, begin by allowing your eyes to focus on the center of the image before slowly expanding your vision and moving outward to include other aspects of the image.

---

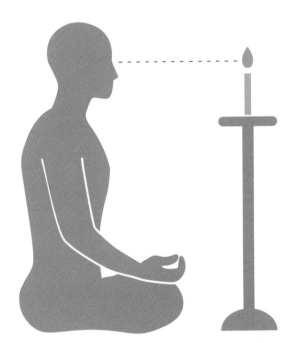

Candle gazing helps you to develop focus and enter into a meditative state.

## TECHNIQUE

1. For this practice, you'll need to be in a darkened room. Light a candle and place it at eye level, approximately 1 yard (1 m) in front of your seat.

2. Sit in any position that's comfortable for you, and begin to settle your body. Release and relax any tension in your muscles. Let your lower body sink toward the floor, and cease any extra or unnecessary movements, such as fidgeting or scratching.

3. Move your attention to the process of breathing. Enjoy three full, conscious breaths, then let your breathing settle into a natural rhythm. Allow the breath to breathe itself.

4. Now focus your gaze on the candle's flame. Try to focus your gaze and minimize blinking. When thoughts arise and cause your mind to wander from the candle, simply let the thoughts go, and gently return your awareness to the flame.

5. Continue to focus on the flame for 5 to 10 minutes, until your eyes begin to water. Then close your eyes, but keep the impression or afterimage of the flame in your mind's eye, and focus your awareness on it. If it's difficult to visualize the afterimage or if it quickly loses clarity, open your eyes and gaze at the candle again for a minute or two, then close your eyes and refocus on the afterimage.

6. When the afterimage fades and you are ready to complete your practice, return your awareness to your breath. Observe the flow of your breath for a minute before opening your eyes.

---

Meditation practices that use an anchor for the mind are among the most widely studied. Anchors have been found to activate the brain's frontal cortex, which is involved in optimizing attention, focus, memory, language, judgment, problem solving, and impulse control. Enhanced activity in this area explains why meditators are less easily distracted, are more focused, and show greater speed and accuracy when performing tasks.

The frontal cortex is also the area of the brain that's largely responsible for our higher and more complex faculties, such as social and moral reasoning. It enables us to plan and think ahead, and to engage in complex decision-making processes. Essentially, it's the home of our conscious, considered, aware self. Meditation-induced activity in the frontal lobes correlates with positive changes in emotional and psychological well-being.

---

## ⬤ PRACTICE TIPS

Formal Practice: Practice daily for 10 to 20 minutes.

# 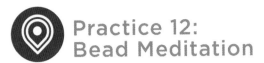 Practice 12: Bead Meditation

Bead meditations can be found in spiritual traditions throughout the world, and they include the Roman Catholic rosary, the Hindu *japa mala*, the Buddhist *mala*, and the Muslim *mishbaha*. Each involves the use of a string of beads as a focus for the mind and body during meditation, as the meditator recites a mantra or prayer (or simply observes the breath) while proceeding bead by bead through the string.

Traditions differ in terms of the number of beads found on the string, the materials the beads are made from, which hand and fingers are used to work the beads, where the hands are placed on the body, and the recitations that are spoken or chanted as the worshipper progresses along the string. For example, the *mishbaha* contains 99 beads; the *japa mala* has 108, and the rosary contains five sets of 10 small beads separated by another larger bead. There is generally a "head," "guru," or "parent" bead of a different size, which serves the practical purpose of designating the starting point for the circuit. Many systems recite a prayer either silently or aloud or use a devotional phrase or mantra while moving the beads through the fingers.

The hands can be held at different locations on the body, including the lap or the knee, or they can be suspended 1 inch (2.5 cm) or so in front of the heart or navel. Although the beads are most commonly held in one hand, some traditions use both hands. The Hindu *mala* is typically held in the right hand, and the index finger is explicitly avoided. In contrast, Buddhist and Catholic traditions do not follow this rule, and the beads may be held in either hand and worked through any finger. Ultimately, unless you're explicitly committed to a particular tradition, there are no fixed rules regarding the "right" way to use beads for meditation. Here's how to begin your practice.

## TECHNIQUE

1. Sit in any position that's comfortable for you. Hold your string of beads in one hand and close your eyes.

2. Begin by gently moving your attention to the process of breathing. Enjoy three full, conscious breaths and then let your breath settle into a natural rhythm. Allow the breath to breathe itself.

3. Drape the string of beads over one of your fingers and use the thumb to slide the string, allowing you to move from one bead to the next. Move the thumb in an inward direction, pulling the beads toward you.

4. Start with the "head" bead, then move to the next one, and begin to recite your mantra either aloud or silently, or rest your awareness on your breath. One bead can represent each cycle of breath. If you're reciting a prayer or multiword mantra, recite the entire mantra on each bead (instead of using one bead per word). If you get distracted or lose your focus during this process, simply return to the bead you were on and pick up from there. (Getting distracted is perfectly normal, so try not to judge yourself!)

5. Continue reciting the mantra with each bead until you return to the "head" bead, then pause, mentally and physically. (The "head" bead isn't counted as part of the circuit.) If you're continuing, flip the string of beads around and start again.

### ⬤ PRACTICE TIP

Practice daily for 10 to 20 minutes.

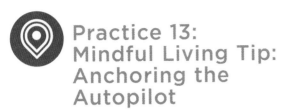

## Practice 13: Mindful Living Tip: Anchoring the Autopilot

Throughout this chapter, you've been cultivating your ability to settle your mind using an anchor. Now it's time to bring this kind of stable, conscious, meditative awareness to your day-to-day activities to help you break the habit of autopilot.

Autopilot isn't a bad thing altogether. It's actually an amazing adaptive feature of the human brain, and it allows us to do and manage several things at once. It allows the brain to simplify an incredibly complex activity, like driving a car, into an easily executed repertoire of behaviors that require little mental effort. But autopilot has gone too far when we start missing out on actually experiencing life because of it.

### LIST OF REPETITIVE ACTIVITIES

| | |
|---|---|
| Cutting vegetables | Shaving |
| Cleaning | Brushing hair |
| Painting | Laundry |
| Lawn mowing | Knitting |
| Gardening | Running |
| Walking | Stroking a pet |

### STEP 1

Choose an activity during which you typically shift into autopilot, such as shaving, jogging, or any of the repetitive daily tasks in the box to the left.

### STEP 2

Next time you're engaged in this activity, try to bring your awareness completely to the task at hand. Awaken your senses and pay attention to the movements the task requires and to the sensations that result from it. For example, if you're folding laundry, notice the texture of the fabric. Lift the sheets or towels to your nose and explore their scent. Consider the weight of different items—socks, T-shirts, blankets, pillowcases—and observe the fine movements of your fingers and hands as you fold and stack. When your mind wanders, be patient with yourself, and move your awareness back to the task at hand.

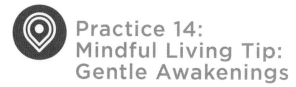

# Practice 14:
# Mindful Living Tip:
# Gentle Awakenings

Waking gradually is one of the simplest, gentlest mindfulness practices we can bring to the start of each and every day. It sets the tone for the day ahead and allows us to consciously experience deep timelessness before the clock-time begins.

There's no precise formula for creating a gentle awakening routine, and I've found that meditators tend to craft their own routines based on their favorite practices. Here are some tips for getting your practice underway:

- **Breathe.** Begin your day by stepping into the stream of your breath. There's no need to change anything after all, your breath has breathed you all night long. Simply stay in bed and savor the simple pleasure of bringing mindfulness to your breath.

- **Be grateful.** This day is a gift, a gift that has already been given to you. One day—far from now, hopefully—you won't receive this gift: but for today, it's all yours.

- **Feel your body.** A quick body scan from head to toe is all it takes to become resident in your physical form. Check in with your physical body and, if you wish, flood each area with gratitude and love as you become aware of it.

- **Scope the landscape.** Check out the internal landscape of your body and mind. Notice any sensations and any emotions. Do you feel warm or cold? Rested or still sleepy? Does that dream you're just waking from still seem very real to you? You don't need to do anything about these physical and emotional states—just notice them for now.

- **First encounters.** Be especially mindful during the first encounters of your day. These moments might involve other people or they might not. Your first encounters may be with yourself, as you shower, make coffee, or get dressed. Either way, bring total presence and awareness to these moments.

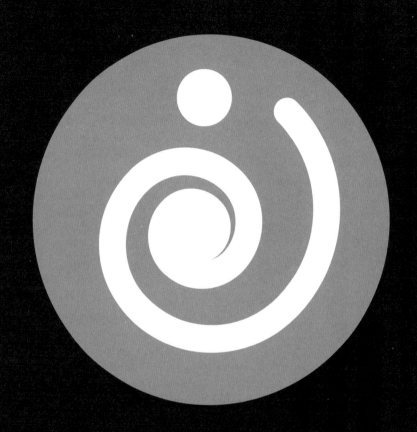

:: CHAPTER 4 ::

# WAKING THE WITNESS

IN THE LAST CHAPTER, YOU LEARNED THAT HAVING AN ANCHOR FOR THE MIND CAN BE HELPFUL FOR CALMING MENTAL ACTIVITY AND FOR BRINGING A SENSE OF REST AND PEACE TO BOTH BODY AND MIND. BUT WHETHER YOU'RE A NEW OR AN EXPERIENCED MEDITATOR, YOU PROBABLY NOTICED THAT YOUR MIND DRIFTED INTO THINKING, REGARDLESS OF WHICH TYPE OF ANCHOR YOU USED (BREATH, MANTRA, OR OBJECT). YOU'LL PROBABLY ALSO HAVE NOTICED THAT, AS YOU CONTINUED TO PRACTICE, YOU WERE ABLE TO GENTLY REDIRECT YOUR ATTENTION BACK TO THE ANCHOR. SO THE QUESTION IS THIS: WHEN YOUR MIND WAS MEANDERING, WHO WAS IT THAT NOTICED AND REACTED? WHO DREW YOUR AWARENESS BACK TO THE ANCHOR SO PATIENTLY BUT PERSISTENTLY? WHO WAS WATCHING THE ENTIRE PROCESS AND OVERSEEING IT WHEN YOUR MIND HAD WANDERED AWAY?

The answer, of course, is you. You were the only participant in your experience. You were simultaneously focusing your mind and overseeing the process of focusing your mind. You redirected your awareness when it drifted.

Incredible, isn't it? How were you able to be absorbed in thinking while also being aware enough to choose a response? Here's how: There's a part of you that wasn't swept away with your thoughts and feelings. An aspect of your being was aware of them, but it wasn't fused or identified with them. This is known as either your "observing self" or your "witnessing self." In psychology, this process is known as metacognition and it's an important skill to cultivate—both for meditation and for daily life.

In this chapter, then, you'll dive deeper into the nature of the witnessing mind, and you'll learn practices that have been designed to help you cultivate your ability to become the watcher, or witness, of your own mind.

# ⓘ KEY CONCEPT: METACOGNITION

**Metacognition** is the process of reflecting on your own mental processes. It is the act of thinking about thinking: and the experience of being aware of awareness.

In meditation, we begin to notice that we are noticing. We start to look *at* our thoughts rather than *from* our thoughts, and in doing so, we develop and strengthen the skill of metacognition. We learn to see thoughts for what they are—just thoughts. We learn to see mind stuff for what it is—just transient mind stuff. We become aware that our identities consist of much more than just our busy thinking minds, and we become more able to resist unhelpful and negative patterns of thinking.

In a way, metacognition and meditation practices strengthen our psychological immune system by gradually exposing us to thoughts, distractions, and physical sensations as we train ourselves not to react to them. Over time, we begin to become more objective toward these things, and we see them for what they are—transient, impermanent mental events.

The development of metacognition also highlights one of the key differences between meditation and relaxation: Relaxation tools are designed to release stress and tension from the body, while meditation techniques also train the mind to be less reactive. This explains why mindfulness has emerged as a powerful, evidence-based tool for enhancing psychological health, especially for those with clinical disorders like anxiety, depression, and substance abuse. It's been shown to not only improve overall mood—thus lessening the likelihood of experiencing negative and unhelpful thoughts—but it also helps us cope with these types of thoughts when they do arise. Research indicates that, through meditation, we can become less reactive to such thoughts, and can handle them with greater ease and composure.

---

**Metacognition** is defined as "cognition about cognition" or "knowing about knowing." More simply, it's the ability to think about your own processes of thinking. Meditation both requires and cultivates this skill.

---

# THOUGHTS ON THINKING

It's a common and dangerous misconception that thoughts must be overcome in meditation or that the goal of meditation is a thought-free mind. The truth is that, though there are states of consciousness or awareness in which it seems that the mind has finally stopped chattering, thoughts will soon begin again. That's part of being human. Meditation is not a thought-eradication device. But it *does* enable us to disengage from mental chatter (without insisting that the mental chatter stop completely) and "drop" into a much more expansive space of being.

Remember that resisting thoughts is essentially the same as indulging them. Trying to control your thoughts with other thoughts is probably the longest and most difficult route to a better relationship with your own mind. So avoid getting stuck in this trap. After all, no one can command the mind to stop thinking any more than you can command your heart to stop beating. That said, though, we *can* train both our hearts and our minds to benefit our well-being. We train the heart through cardiovascular exercise—like walking, jogging, running, or swimming—and we train the mind through meditation.

During meditation, we learn to see thoughts for exactly what they are—no more and no less. That doesn't mean that we cease to be thinking beings, but we do become less reactive to that internal dialogue. We learn to detach from it when we wish to, and we spend less time ruminating, or going over and over the same thing in our heads. Plus, we suffer less. We enjoy a greater sense of clarity. It's true that, as a result of meditation, we begin to experience gaps between our thoughts—not by suppressing or avoiding them, but rather by accepting yet moving beyond them.

**"Your goal is not to battle with the mind, but to witness the mind."**

**—SWAMI MUKTANANDA**

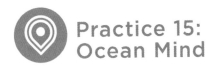

## Practice 15: Ocean Mind

The witnessing aspect of awareness is like the ocean. Your thoughts and your shifting moods and sensations are like waves on the ocean's surface. Some days, the swell of the waves is full, heaving, and relentless; Their rhythm is strong, turbulent, and pounding. On other days, the surface of the ocean may seem like a lake with delicate waves that lap gently at the shore's edge. No matter how big or small the waves are, they all share a common characteristic: they arise, and then they pass away. They also take place within a much larger context—the ocean—and they emerge from that expansive space to reach a peak before they break and disappear back into the ocean's depths.

How do we approach these waves? We can't stop them from coming, but we can learn to surf on and with them. We can learn to ride them out, and we can also learn to dive beneath them. Imagine for a moment that you are diving to the very bottom of the ocean. Down there, the current is so gentle that it's nearly nonexistent. From this deep stillness, you can cast your eyes back up toward the surface of the ocean where the ever-changing pattern of waves continues to unfold. You can see the movement on the surface without being caught up in it. You can rest in the vast peace below the surface of the ocean while allowing the shifting, changing activity to carry on up above.

Our witnessing mind is like the ocean's depths. It is the realm of our being that holds the space in which all of our life experiences can arise and pass away. Our thoughts, feelings, and sensations are like the ever-changing surface of the ocean. Whether they're stormy or placid, the deeper expanse of the ocean beneath always remains the same—vast, unaffected, and clear.

Meditation can be a choppy, blustery affair when we first begin to practice. Thoughts arise again and again, like tempestuous waves, and they just keep on coming. Our minds move in all directions, like water, and we seem to be thinking more than meditating. In fact, there's even more *stuff* in our minds than there was before, and focusing it feels impossible. Could meditation be causing us to think *more*, rather than less? Not at all. Relax and rest assured that nothing has changed. Your mind is as it was before you began meditating; you're just more aware of it now.

Know that things will eventually settle down. True, the thought waves keep coming, but with time and practice, we learn to ride them and dive beneath them. They might come in sets, followed by still gaps in between—but we begin to know and perceive all of them as temporary passing events. Then a moment arrives at which the ocean becomes more like a lake. Gentle ripples of passing thoughts touch the shore. Moments of stillness occur, and then another storm blows in.

That's natural. Experienced meditators tell us that the surface of the ocean doesn't transform into an infinitely still lake, even after many years of practice. Buddhist nun Pema Chödrön, for instance, is a wonderful source of encouragement, humility, and practical advice on this concept. She assures us that, even after four decades as a full-time meditator, she still experiences thoughts during meditation. She may be experienced, but she's human, after all, and one of the functions of the human mind is to think.

Yes, even when you've become a practiced meditator, some thoughts may still hook you, trip you up, and toss you around more than others—particularly when you're facing certain stressors in life. At other times, you'll be able to sit back and see the chaos for what it is. You'll surf those waves instead of getting pounded onto the shore, and, even in the murkiest, most chaotic moments, you'll remember that *you are the ocean* and not just the waves. You can swim to the bottom and, amidst the stillness, watch the wild dance unfolding on the surface above.

## TECHNIQUE

1.  Sit in any position that's comfortable for you and close your eyes.

2.  Begin by gently moving your attention to the process of breathing. Enjoy three full, slow, deep breaths. Fill the abdomen as you inhale and allow your entire body to soften as you exhale. Then allow your breath to settle into a natural rhythm. Let the breath breathe you.

3.  Choose from either your breath or mantra meditation practice (see chapter 3), and gently rest your awareness on your chosen anchor.

4.  You'll inevitably find your mind wandering, caught by distracting thoughts, external experiences, or bodily sensations. When you notice this, pause for a moment and acknowledge the witnessing part of your mind that has noticed the wandering thoughts. Allow this witnessing mind to watch and observe what's happening at the surface of your mind.

5.  Imagine your witnessing self as the restful depths of the ocean. From this space of stillness, look back up and toward the ever-changing surface of the ocean, where thoughts, like waves, arise and pass away. View wandering thoughts as temporary waves on the surface of the ocean.

6. Now use your anchor to move your awareness back to the depths of the ocean. Your job is not to judge your thoughts, engage in a battle with them, or create a thought-free mind. Remember that thoughts are not problems; they are an essential part of meditation. Your practice is to notice thoughts, refrain from fusing or identifying with them, let them go, and gently redirect your awareness to your anchor.

7. At the end of your practice, take a few moments to expand your awareness from the breath into the room around you. When you feel ready, open your eyes.

## ○ PRACTICE TIP

Formal Practice: Aim to practice this meditation for 12 to 20 minutes daily.

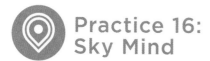

## Practice 16: Sky Mind

The sky is another powerful analogy that can help you understand the witnessing aspect of your awareness. Imagine that your thoughts are like clouds in the sky; they're always changing, and they arise and pass away continuously. Sometimes, there are big, heavy, gray clouds that linger; other times there are hardly any clouds at all. Sometimes, the clouds move swiftly, and other times they seem to hang overhead. Here's the interesting part: Different kinds of clouds may blow in, but the sky that holds them remains exactly the same, untouched and ever present. The sky doesn't anticipate future clouds or chase after visible ones. It simply observes the unfolding and ever-changing display of clouds as they arise and pass away. The sky remains an ever-clear, perfect presence—just like your witnessing mind.

In this exercise, you'll learn to cultivate the skill of metacognition through the technique of **noting**, which involves softly labeling your mind stuff. For example, when you're observing a thought, you might like to use the generic label "mind stuff" or "thinking." You could also become more attuned to the type of mind stuff that has distracted you, such as "memory," "worry," "fantasy," or "planning."

This noting technique is particularly helpful when you find yourself really caught up in a particular thought or set of thoughts. It enables you to distance yourself from the thought so that you can redirect your awareness to your meditation anchor and your witnessing mind. It's best conceptualized as an aid, like training wheels on a bicycle. It can be very helpful, but it should be used sparingly, and the ultimate goal is to continue on without it.

---

The **noting** technique involves applying a one-word label, such as "thinking," "hearing," or "worry," to whatever arises in your mind.

---

### TECHNIQUE

1. Sit in any position that's comfortable for you and close your eyes.

2. Begin by gently moving your attention to the process of breathing. Enjoy three full, slow, deep breaths. Fill the abdomen as you inhale and allow your entire body to soften as you exhale. Then allow your breath to settle into a natural rhythm. Let the breath breathe you.

3. Choose from either your breath or mantra meditation practice (see chapter 3), and gently rest your awareness on your chosen anchor.

4. You'll inevitably find your mind wandering, caught by distracting thoughts, external experiences, or bodily sensations. When you notice this, pause for a moment and acknowledge the witnessing part of your mind that has noticed the wandering thoughts. Imagine your witnessing self as the sky, vast and expansive. From this space, look toward your ever-changing, wandering

thoughts as if they were passing clouds. Allow this witnessing mind to watch and observe what's happening at the surface of the mind.

5. Begin to use the noting technique. Label your surface thinking as "mind stuff" or "thinking," or label them more specifically according to the "type" of the thinking they represent (for example, "memory" or "planning"). Gently, but firmly, label the thought without judgment. Let it be, but let it go, and keep returning your awareness to your anchor. Your job is not to judge your thoughts, engage in a battle with them, or create a thought-free mind. Remember that thoughts are not problems; they are an essential part of meditation. Your practice is to notice thoughts, refrain from fusing or identifying with them, let them go, and gently redirect your awareness to your anchor.

6. At the end of your practice, take a few moments to expand your awareness from the breath into the room around you. When you feel ready, open your eyes.

## ○ PRACTICE TIP

Formal Practice: Aim to practice this meditation for 12 to 20 minutes daily.

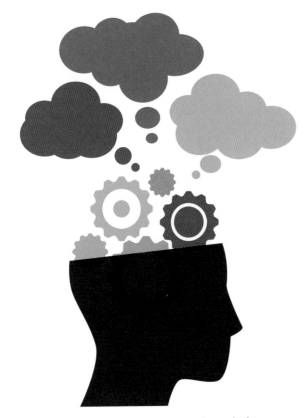

Let your busy thoughts go and watch them float away like clouds.

## Practice 17: Mindful Living Tip: The Commentator

Developing metacognition—the witnessing mind—is a powerful practice that can help bring greater calm and clarity to your daily life. Your formal meditation practice is your training ground, but your daily life is the area in which your new skills are really tested, and where those skills can bring you great benefit. That's why it's important to approach meditation as a dynamic activity that you weave into your day-to-day life. Meditation isn't limited to the 20 minutes per day you spend on your meditation cushion!

We typically move through our days awash in a river of thoughts, sensations, and emotions, and sometimes we can feel like a rudderless ship at the mercy of the weather. We are tossed about—and often swept away—by whichever thoughts and feelings are prominent at the moment. Wouldn't it be wonderful to get some distance from these events while they're happening? That's far more useful that demanding that they stop—because we simply *can't* force them to stop. Life is an ever-changing flow of experiences. But we can learn to detach from, or "dis-identify," with them. We can develop the ability to become less caught up in them, and you've already been cultivating this skill throughout chapter 4.

Here are some further ways to cultivate greater metacognition and your "witnessing self" by becoming more aware of your own mind as you go about your day-to-day activities:

- When you are performing an action, awaken an internal commentator to observe (without judgment) what you're doing. For example, as you're walking to work in the morning, say to yourself, "I am walking." When you're washing the dinner dishes, say, "I'm washing the dishes."

- Allow the commentator to also observe what your *mind* is doing, especially when it has drifted away from the task at hand. For example, when you find yourself ruminating over an argument you had with a colleague, you could say to yourself, "Thinking about the argument with Sarah," or you could label the type of thought process as "remembering," "rehashing," or "ruminating." Or, if your witnessing self notices that you're feeling full of love toward your child, partner, or friend, you can articulate this by saying to yourself, "Feeling love for Thomas." Simply make a mental note of what your mind is doing.

- Take a few moments throughout the day to pause and observe your mind. Is it in the present moment, or is it somewhere in the past or future? There's no right or wrong here—just observe. For example, you might be in the act of watering a plant, but when you witness your mind, you might notice that your mind isn't watering the plant at all—it's planning what to make for dinner instead. Make a mental note of this, or label it as "planning dinner." Enjoy the spacious pause that occurs when you watch your mind instead of remaining immersed within it. Then, make a conscious choice and decide whether you'd like to continue planning dinner or redirect your awareness to the present moment in which you're watering your plant.

- This kind of commentary is a tool to help you enhance your ability to detach from thoughts. But it's got nothing to do with changing your experience. The witnessing mind notices and allows every aspect of life to enter it and leave. It does not judge, evaluate, grasp, or refuse any experience. Its attitude is one of allowance—and curiosity, too.

- Performing this kind of mental commentary might feel weird to you—and let's be honest, it is kind of weird. After all, you wouldn't want to distance yourself from *all* your experiences because you're so busy commentating to yourself on them. At the same time, though, you wouldn't want to spend every moment of every day at the whim of your mind, unable to get some much-needed distance from transient emotions and thought processes. So, think of the commentator as a tool to use to enhance your metacognitive awareness and to strengthen your ability to remain centered in the midst of thought storms. Use it, practice it, and certainly return to it as needed—but you'll probably find that it's best not to spend entire days being a commentator upon your own life.

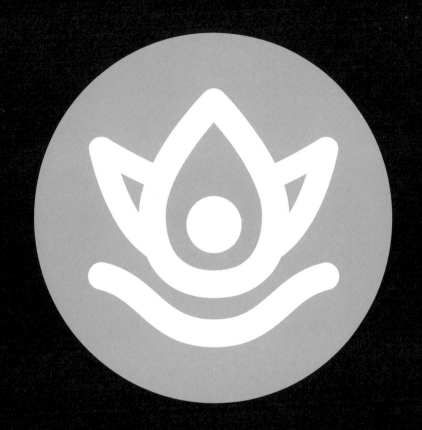

:: CHAPTER 5 ::

# OPENING TO PRESENCE

JUST AS YOU CAN TRAIN YOUR BODY THROUGH PHYSICAL EXERCISE, SO TOO CAN YOU TRAIN YOUR MIND THROUGH THE PRACTICE OF MEDITATION. IN THE LAST FEW CHAPTERS, YOU'VE BEEN DEVELOPING YOUR MIND'S ABILITY TO REMAIN SETTLED AND STABLE IN THE FACE OF DISTRACTIONS, AND TO DO THIS YOU'VE USED OBJECTS SUCH AS THE BREATH, A MANTRA, OR AN IMAGE SUCH AS AN ANCHOR. IN CHAPTER 4, YOU EXPLORED WAYS TO DEVELOP YOUR METACOGNITIVE AWARENESS—THAT IS, YOUR ABILITY TO BE AWARE OF YOUR OWN THINKING INSTEAD OF BEING CAUGHT UP IN IT. HERE, IN CHAPTER 5, YOU'LL EXTEND THAT TRAINING. YOU'LL EXPLORE TECHNIQUES THAT CULTIVATE AWARENESS OF AWARENESS ITSELF—AS WELL AS YOUR ABILITY TO HOLD YOUR AWARENESS IN THE PRESENT MOMENT.

These practices are known as **open awareness** meditations. They're a bit different from the techniques you've explored in the preceding chapters in that they don't ask you to use an object to anchor your mind. Instead, you'll learn to use the ever-changing nature of your experience as the focus for your awareness. During this practice, you'll simply be open, awake, and alert to whatever arises within the internal and external landscape of your experience. (The internal landscape encompasses your thoughts, feelings, and physical sensations, while the external landscape contains all that you can perceive with your five senses.) It's all about developing your capacity to be present to whatever arises in your life experience, retaining the element of gracious mindful awareness, but without focusing on any specific object.

There are several approaches to open awareness meditation. It's commonly practiced in Theravadin Buddhist traditions, the spiritual lineage that has profoundly influenced the mindfulness movement and has shaped the way in which the majority of Westerners encounter meditation today. open awareness is taught

**Open awareness** meditations cultivate a kind of panoramic awareness of whatever is happening in the present moment without the use of a specific focus or anchor for the mind. These types of practices are also called open monitoring and nondirective meditations.

in Dzogchen, an advanced Tibetan Buddhist practice in which meditators are encouraged to turn their attention toward the awareness that is attending. In the Zen tradition, this approach is called "the backward step," since it encourages us to step out and away from our common routine of engaging with all experiences in the foreground of life (like sights, sounds, and thoughts) and step into the background presence, or the space from which all these things arise.

In most traditional contexts, these open awareness practices are taught after a student has become familiar with settling and stabilizing the mind using an anchor such as the breath or mantra (see chapter 3). While it is certainly possible for beginners to start with open awareness practices, many people find that they're easily swept away by thoughts and emotional reactions when they haven't had a chance to develop their capacity to stabilize their attention. If you're a beginner and this happens to you as you try to rest in pure awareness, it might be a good idea to revisit some of the practices in chapter 3 before you continue.

## ❶ KEY CONCEPT: NONJUDGMENT

Nonjudgment means being open and impartial to our experiences. It clears the pathway for new perspectives and greater wisdom. Observing our own thoughts without judgment gives us an opportunity to begin to notice the editing, analyzing, and intellectualizing aspects of our minds. This means we can cultivate greater awareness and intentionality in our day-to-day lives.

Nonjudgment isn't easy for many of us, and in some ways, it's like swimming upstream against strong evolutionary hardwiring. Our brains are judgment machines, hardwired (and trained) to compare and contrast, to like or dislike, and

### SPOTLIGHT ON SCIENCE

Open awareness meditation techniques may be useful for chronic pain sufferers. Studies show that these meditations are characterized by a greater presence of theta- and gamma-wave brain activity, and they're also reported to be beneficial for cultivating creativity in comparison with the focused mindfulness of breath meditation (see Practice 9).

to judge things as good or bad, important or not important. And that's okay. Cultivating the quality of nonjudgment doesn't mean that judgment is bad. It's not. It's just that we tend to judge so quickly that all of our experiences become colored by past events and old standpoints. As a result, we can miss out on fresh perspectives and experiencing life in new ways.

In mindfulness meditation, the concept, quality, and attitude of nonjudgment doesn't require you to eradicate your preferences and opinions. You can rest assured that all meditators—including the most practiced ones—still have them, and so will you. It's simply the nature of the body-mind to prefer some experiences over others. But the practice of mindfulness prevents us from being at the mercy of such conditioning, and keeps us from getting swept up in it. That way, we can make more skillful choices. That's why it's important for us to recognize when our minds have entered into the terrain of judgment and analysis. At such moments, all you need to do is be aware of what's happening. (There's no need to complicate things by judging yourself for judging!) Simply recognize the judgment as judgment; gently unhook yourself from its storyline; allow it to play on in the background, if it must; and continue to follow the instructions of your meditation practice.

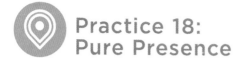

## Practice 18: Pure Presence

The pure presence practice provides a gentle inroad into open awareness meditation. Remember that there's no need to be alarmed if your mind seems to wander more than usual as you begin these new techniques. That's normal, since, instead of resting your mind on an anchor, this practice asks you to stay present to whatever arises without focusing on any specific object.

### TECHNIQUE

1. Sit in any position that's comfortable for you and close your eyes.

2. Begin by gently moving your attention to the process of breathing. Enjoy three full, slow, deep breaths, noticing the movement of your torso and the sound of your breath. Then let your breath settle into a natural rhythm.

3. Now set your mind free. Let it roam and wander. It will soon become aware of something, perhaps a thought, sound, or physical sensation. For instance, you might find yourself thinking of picking up your daughter from her music lesson later in the afternoon, you might hear the central heating turning on, or you might feel a ray of sunlight falling on your right hand. That's fine. Be attentive to whatever comes up without grasping onto anything. Let go of

whatever you notice as soon as it appears in your awareness. Notice and let go—and as you do so, become aware of the awareness that lies underneath your thoughts.

4. Try to remain alert yet relaxed, clear, and aware; you're not fixed on any particular thing, but you're not distracted, either. Without modifying or changing thoughts, feelings, or bodily sensations, allow all things to be just as they are. View all appearances and all experiences as perfectly equal, without liking or disliking or judging anything as better or worse. Maybe your next-door neighbor has started to practice the violin; notice the sound and then release it. Perhaps you notice the lingering scent of your own perfume or cologne. Maybe your stomach is grumbling a little. Whatever it is, observe it, then let it go. If you do find that you're getting caught up in analysis or judgment of these experiences, don't give yourself a hard time. Simply observe these thoughts, then take a breath and redirect your attention to your current experience as it is, toward the awareness that underlies your entire experience.

5. Imagine all thoughts, feelings, and external objects as transitory objects that float past your awareness. Imagine your awareness as a mirror that simply notices and reflects whatever appears in front of it—without clinging, clutching, judging, or indulging.

6. Rest in the sense of spaciousness that arises when the mind ceases to grasp at or resist any experience. This spaciousness can feel incredibly free and expansive—but if you're a beginner, don't worry if your mind starts to wander within a few seconds. That's completely normal. Gently, but persistently, guide your awareness back to the meditation instructions when you notice that this has happened. Remain relaxed and alert within this state of pure reflectivity and equanimity.

7. At the end of your practice, take a few moments to expand your awareness from the breath into the room around you. Become aware of the sounds and scents around you; become aware of your body. Gently wiggle your fingers and toes. When you feel ready, open your eyes.

## ⬥ PRACTICE TIP

Formal Practice: Practice daily for 10 to 20 minutes.

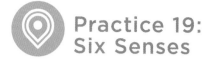

# Practice 19: Six Senses

The six senses practice builds upon the five senses grounding technique from chapter 2 by adding an extra element: the awareness of awareness itself. You'll learn to use the traditional five senses as gateways to explore the present moment and then to enter into the spaciousness that exists when you allow all of these senses to be open, awake, alive, and aware at the same time.

## TECHNIQUE

1. Sit in any position that's comfortable for you and close your eyes.

2. Begin by gently moving your attention to the process of breathing. Enjoy three full, slow, deep breaths, noticing the movement of your torso and the sound of your breath. Then let your breath settle into a natural rhythm.

3. Bring your attention to everything you hear. Notice the sounds around you. First, take note of the loudest, or most prominent, sound you can detect. Then begin to observe all of the quieter sounds in your immediate environment—perhaps even sounds within your own body. Notice them with an attitude of nonjudgmental openness and curiosity.

4. Now shift your attention and focus all of your awareness on everything you can smell. (If you can't smell anything, that's okay. Remember, "no experience" is still an experience.) Explore your sense of smell, but do so without analysis. Simply be wide open to the sheer sensory discovery. Here, there is no such thing as "good" or "bad."

5. Shift your attention and focus all of your awareness on everything you can taste. Your own breath, perhaps? The residue of the chewing gum you tossed out just before you began your practice? The acidic or alkaline taste of your own saliva? Simply notice, without analysis.

6. Now shift your attention and focus all of your awareness on everything you can feel with your skin. Maybe you sense the warmth of sunlight, the prickle of goose bumps, or the way the tag on the back of your shirt is tickling your neck. Do so with a welcoming attitude of nonjudgmental openness and curiosity.

7. Now shift your attention and focus all of your awareness on everything you see behind your eyelids. (Keep your eyes closed.) Be wide open to whatever you experience— pinpoints of light, bursts or washes of color, or sheer blackness.

8. Turn your attention back toward your own mind, toward your sixth sense—that is, metacognition, or the awareness of your own thinking. In your mind's eye, open the backs of your eyes and your inner ears by imagining them. See how they, too, turn inward with intent and awareness. Observe mind stuff arising and passing away.

9. Become a watcher of thoughts. They may be rushing past, like a fast, powerful river, or they might be trickling, like a gentle stream. Perhaps there's space between thoughts, or maybe there's a still and silent backdrop behind them—or not. Simply watch your own mind. Your own experience, whatever it is, is perfectly valid.

10. Now become aware of the you who's watching your mind. Become aware of awareness itself. Be aware of the sense of awareness from which you have observed your own mind. Curiously notice the undercurrent of awareness. Be conscious of your own presence.

11. Let your awareness encompass all of your senses at once: sounds, smells, tastes, textures, sights, and the mind itself—awareness itself. Don't worry if that doesn't last for very long. It's completely normal to have a sense of the "whole" of these experiences, only to have that moment crumble. Simply keep opening yourself to experiencing all of your senses at once, again and again. Allow the experiences of life to continue to unfold in the foreground as you maintain a sense of the alert inner stillness in the background.

12. Can you sense how the experiences of this world continue to play through you, without in any way capturing or confining the inherent spaciousness of awareness? You are the sky with the birds flying through it; you are utterly awake, utterly open. You are awareness itself. Notice this awareness.

13. At the end of your practice, take a few moments to expand your awareness from your breath into the room around you. Become aware of the sounds and scents around you; become aware of your body. Gently wiggle your fingers and toes. When you feel ready, open your eyes.

## ⬤ PRACTICE TIP
Formal Practice: Practice daily for 10 to 20 minutes.

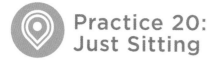

# Practice 20: Just Sitting

*Shikantaza*, which translates as "just sitting," is a type of open awareness meditation practiced in Zen Buddhism. Zen traditions are schools of Buddhism that developed throughout Japan and China, and Zen teachings often circumvent traditional orthodoxy with a kind of radical directness that's designed to cut straight to the point—and the heart—of the lesson.

There is no object to anchor the mind in the practice of *shikantaza*. Instead, the object of the meditation is the space of nonthinking itself. As with previous practices, it's important to note that this space of "nonthinking" is not reached by ignoring the mind or by demanding that it stop its flow of thoughts. Paradoxically, it's reached by letting your awareness glide gently over everything your mind experiences, without attaching or clinging to any of it. In other words, nonthinking is achieved by noticing and letting go.

Don't worry if you find these open awareness practices a little tricky. Lots of people find that their mind seems to wander more during open awareness practices than during other meditations, but that's not really a problem. Remember that it's normal for your mind to run riot—as long as *you're* not running riot with

it. The purpose of meditation isn't to become a world champion at focusing on one thing or on focusing on no-thing. It's about refraining from attaching to thoughts and feelings, and learning not to get caught up in or swept away by them. In many ways, it's about observing, understanding, and dancing with the nature of the mind rather than being at its mercy.

## TECHNIQUE

1. Sit in any position that's comfortable for you and close your eyes.

2. Begin by gently moving your attention to the process of breathing. Enjoy three full, slow, deep breaths. Then let your breath settle into a natural rhythm. Allow the breath to breathe itself.

3. Let go of any effort to focus, and simply leave your mind alone. You'll soon notice that your mind starts to chatter. It might start to show you tempting and pleasurable things—reminiscing about your first kiss as a teenager or anticipating the delicious homemade pizza you're planning to make for dinner—and, like a puppy, your mind might begin to run toward these tantalizing things, but try not to chase them. You don't need to try to get rid of pleasurable thoughts; all you need to do is let them be and avoid getting caught up in chasing them. Let them go.

4. Your mind might also present you with problems, stressors, and worries (the state of your bank account, work conflicts, world politics), and you might notice yourself getting sucked into their vortex. This isn't inevitable, though. Instead, let the unsettling thoughts be there with you. Don't worry about how long they're there. Don't try to push them away or hurry them along. Let them be, but let them go.

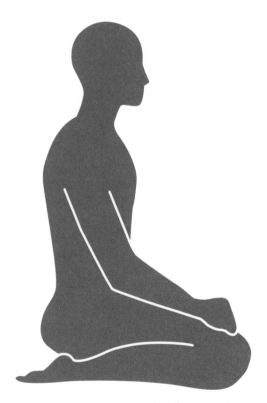

Let your awareness rest in the present moment, exactly as it is.

5. If thoughts are like clouds—arising, taking center stage for a moment, and passing on—then there is also the expanse of sky that surrounds the clouds. Don't worry about actively finding this space. As you continue to allow thoughts to come and go, you will also begin to experience the spaces between them. You don't need to do anything in these empty spaces. Allow yourself to just sit, and be. Relax into nothing. Soon, some kind of mental activity will begin once again. Notice it and let it go. If necessary, return to the breath to center yourself, then keep on letting go of thoughts as they pop up, allowing yourself to enter into the space between thoughts when it presents itself.

6. When you're ready to end your practice, take a few moments to expand your awareness back to your breath and into the room around you. Become aware of the sounds and scents around you; become aware of your body. Gently wiggle your fingers and toes. When you feel ready, open your eyes.

## ⬤ PRACTICE TIP
Formal Practice: Practice daily for 10 to 20 minutes.

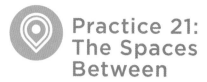

# Practice 21: The Spaces Between

Space is the great container. It is the element and emptiness in which all other elements exist. To the physicist, it is the "field" in which particles move. Some speak of it as "ether," and the ancient yogis called it *akasha*. Although we generally don't pay much attention to the element of space, we've all had experiences in which the space between things has absorbed our attention fully, bringing us into an experience and appreciation of the present moment in a way that the objects within the space could not. For instance, this can happen in our interactions with nature. We might hike to a mountaintop and, from a great height, become aware of the immensity of space, the great chasms and fields of openness surrounding visible things. This perspective is often accompanied by a sense of expansiveness. It shifts us from our everyday, three-dimensional view of the world into a multidimensional, all-encompassing, wide-open state of being.

Now, the question isn't whether we are capable of becoming aware of the spaces between things. We already know that these experiences can and do occur. The question is whether we can cultivate our awareness of space, whether we can train ourselves to drop the rigidity of object-oriented awareness and become more open to the presence of space. Many meditation traditions suggest that we certainly can, and this mind-opening practice will guide you to explore the spaces between things, using your own body as a playground.

Don't feel you have to follow these instructions to the letter. Consider them as invitations to your mind that encourage it to explore new modes of awareness. Because this meditation guides your awareness to the phenomenon of space, you might be tempted to analyze the space in traditional, linear ways—but see if you can guide your awareness to "feel" rather than "think" about your experience. For example, if you're guided to imagine the space between your eyes, try to *feel* into the space rather than using a measurement to imagine it, such as "1 inch" or "1 centimeter." The ideal response is whatever feeling comes to you most naturally. Try to sense your response instead of "thinking" it. Tap into your "feeling mind" rather than your "analytical mind."

## TECHNIQUE

1. Sit in any position that's comfortable for you. Settle your body and close your eyes.

2. Begin by gently moving your attention to the process of breathing. Enjoy three full, conscious breaths. Then allow your breath to settle into a natural rhythm.

3. As you breathe, imagine the space inside your nostrils. Then, traveling through your nostrils, imagine the space behind your eyes.

4. Move from your eyes to the space between your temples, to the volume of space inside your cheeks, and to the volume of space inside your ears. Imagine also the distance between each ear. Imagine the entire region of your head and face, and the volume of space within it.

5. Now imagine the distance between the underside of your chin and your shoulders. Imagine the volume of space within your throat and neck. As you inhale, imagine filling this space with air, and as you exhale, imagine the breath draining from the area, and how it fills with space after the breath has disappeared.

6. Imagine the space inside your lungs. As you inhale, imagine filling this space with air, and as you exhale, imagine the breath draining from the area, and how it fills with space after the breath has disappeared. Imagine the distance between each outer edge of your rib cage, and the space within the rib cage. Imagine your stomach and the volume of space within it. Imagine your organs and the way in which they, too, are permeated by space.

7. Imagine your pelvis, and the space this bony structure contains. Imagine your bones themselves. They might seem to be dense and hard, but they're actually composed of space. Imagine the space within your bones, containing bone marrow. Imagine the spine and the space within vertebrae.

8. Extend your awareness to contemplate your entire body, including your arms, legs, hands, and feet. Imagine the volume of space within you.

9. Imagine now that your whole body is composed of atoms of matter—which, indeed, it is. Since atoms are predominantly composed of space, you, too, are mostly composed of space.

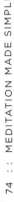

10. Now extend your awareness beyond your body to the room you're in. Consider the space between you and other objects in the room. Imagine the space between the walls. Imagine the space within you and the space surrounding you.

11. When you're ready to end your practice, take a moment to return your awareness back to your breath and into the room around you. Gently wiggle your fingers and toes. Stretch your limbs a little. When you feel ready, open your eyes.

## ⬤ PRACTICE TIP

Formal Practice: Practice daily for 10 to 20 minutes.

### SPOTLIGHT ON SCIENCE

Recent research suggests that open awareness techniques (like those offered here in chapter 5) activate parts of the brain that enhance different kinds of problem-solving skills than those enhanced by meditations that use an anchor (such as those offered in chapter 3).

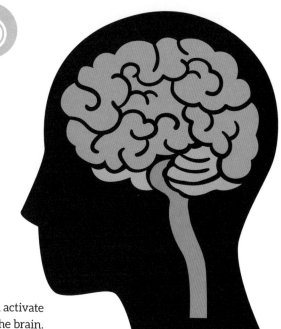

Different types of meditation activate different parts of the brain.

## Practice 22: Mindful Living Tip: Dancing Emptiness

Dancing emptiness is a daily practice for bringing the meditative awareness you developed in Practice 21 (The Spaces Between) to life. It invites you to extend your awareness to notice not only objects themselves, but also the fertile field of space and dancing emptiness that exists between them. If you're wondering how emptiness can "dance," remember that space isn't just a void: it's still kinetic and energized—and powerful, too. This awareness can be immensely helpful in daily life; it can act as a powerful antidote to the kind of narrow vision and "small mind" that accompanies stress. As you probably know all too well, stress doesn't feel expansive. Stress zeros in our attention on our challenges, our suffering, or our problems. And it doesn't notice the spaciousness that's contained within and around all of our experiences. The dancing emptiness practice helps soften the rigid boundaries of this limited way of thinking.

### STEP 1

Wherever you are right now—it doesn't matter whether you're outside or inside—bring your awareness to the space between things. For example, notice the space between your face and this book. Notice the space between your arms, and the distance between your head and feet. Notice the volume of space between your arms.

Now, notice the space between you and an object near to you, such as a piece of furniture or a tree. Extend your perspective to another object near to you, and then to one that's a little farther away. Keep on extending your awareness in this way; enjoy letting your awareness dance in the embrace of space, which is within, around, and between all things.

### STEP 2

Next time you take a mindful pause or enjoy a little breathing space, consider expanding your awareness to the emptiness and spaciousness within and around you. You can experience this within your own body, as we did in Practice 21, or you can do it by noticing the external world, as described in step 1.

# Practice 23: Mindful Living Tip: 3-Minute Mind Shower

By now, you're able to direct your awareness in different ways. You're able to tune in to what's happening in the internal landscape of your body and mind in the present moment (chapters 3 and 4). You've also learned to anchor your awareness and stabilize your mind by placing your attention on one thing—without resisting other distractions, but by simply letting them go (chapter 4). And you've practiced resting in the spaciousness of awareness itself (chapter 5).

Now it's time to draw on these techniques to master the 3-minute mind shower, a quick and effective practice for releasing stress, balancing your nervous system, and refreshing your mind. The best part is, you can use at any time throughout your day.

## MINUTE 1

Let your awareness drop into the present moment as you experience it in your body and mind. Begin by taking at least three full, conscious breaths, then tune in to your awareness with a curious mind and ask yourself, "What are the thoughts, emotions, and sensations present within me in this moment?" Try not to push anything away. Put out a welcome mat for whatever appears.

## MINUTE 2

Choose one aspect of your current experience to anchor your mind, such as your breath, a feeling, a sensation, or a sound. Give it center stage in your awareness. Let all other distractions come and go in the background. Keep on returning your awareness to your anchor, keeping it at the foreground of your attention.

## MINUTE 3

Now rest in awareness itself. Let your entire being rest in the space that perceives all things: awareness itself. Experience this oceanic, sky-like spaciousness. Sit with it and let it fill you completely. Then, take a deep breath and return to your usual activities.

## ⬥ PRACTICE TIP

Visualize an hourglass as you practice; it's the perfect image for the flow of this exercise. Watch the flow of the sand through the hourglass as you move from expansive (Minute 1) to fine-tuned (Minute 2) and back to expansive (Minute 3).

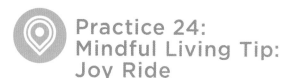

## Practice 24:
## Mindful Living Tip:
## Joy Ride

Joy matters. In a world where stress has reached epidemic proportions for many of us, it's vital not only to manage the causes and symptoms of stress, but also to infuse life with joy. This joy riding exercise takes around 10 minutes to prepare, and only 5 to 10 minutes each day to practice, but it's one of the most powerful practices for bringing more joy and mindfulness into your life.

Write down ten *small* things (that is, things that can be accomplished or achieved on most "regular" days) that make you happy. Try not to aim big, because it's really very important to keep these things small! All of us have larger-scale events or activities that we love, such as traveling or going on family holidays, but the purpose of this joy ride exercise is to uncover life's simple daily pleasures.

Your joy ride list is as unique as you are. Mine includes listening to music, watching the sunrise, and lying on the floor for cuddles with my dog.

### STEP 1

Invest 10 minutes in yourself and write out as many joy ride activities as you can think of. Try not to judge or censor yourself. Don't worry about whether your list seems corny, silly, clichéd, or crazy. It's yours!

### STEP 2

Put your list in a place where you'll see it regularly, like on the fridge or beside your desk at work. Check it each day, and try to complete two of the activities on it. If you're already taking daily joy rides, try diving in deeper: do more than two each day, or add new ones to your list.

### STEP 3

As you enjoy your joy ride, take a pause to soak in the sheer pleasure of the moment. Explore your pleasure more fully by asking yourself:

- What physical sensations can I feel right now?
- What thoughts am I experiencing?
- What feelings are floating to the surface?
- Then watch as your daily joy quota grows.

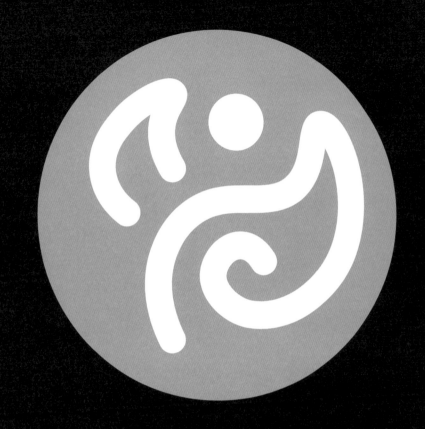

:: CHAPTER 6 ::

# MOVING WITH INTENTION

INSTRUCTIONS FOR BEING IN THE PRESENT MOMENT OFTEN SOUND SO SIMPLE. "WHEN YOU'RE WALKING, JUST WALK," OR "WHEN YOU'RE EATING, EAT." THE TRUTH IS, BRINGING MINDFULNESS TO YOUR DAILY MOVEMENTS AND ACTIONS CAN BE CHALLENGING, BUT THIS CHAPTER IS HERE TO HELP. YOU'LL BEGIN TO EXPLORE TWO TRADITIONAL MOVING MINDFULNESS PRACTICES THAT WILL HELP YOU APPLY WHAT YOU'VE LEARNED SO FAR IN THIS BOOK TO YOUR DAY-TO-DAY LIFE. BECAUSE THEY SOUND SO SIMPLE, YOU MIGHT BE TEMPTED TO PASS THEM BY AND MOVE ON TO OTHER TECHNIQUES. I ENCOURAGE YOU TO TRY THEM AT LEAST ONCE TO SEE IF THEY'RE RIGHT FOR YOU.

## ❶ KEY CONCEPT: BEGINNER'S MIND

The concept of **beginner's mind**, or *shoshin*, has its roots in Zen Buddhism and it describes a way of experiencing life that's unencumbered by past experiences and prior knowledge. It invites us to approach our world as a child does: with curiosity and a sense of wonder and openness to new possibilities.

A beginner's mind is like a clean slate. It is aware that it has never experienced this particular moment before. It involves less expectation and more anticipation. It embraces spontaneity and approaches each moment as if it were its very first. This attitude is a great ally to meditators, and it's something we can cultivate as we practice. Plus, it's an antidote to the automatic pilot mode. It helps us break free of the ingrained assumptions and habitual modes of thinking that often keep us from seeing things as they really are, and it allows us to re-encounter the richness of our experiences. We can bring our beginner's mind to both our meditation practice and our everyday lives.

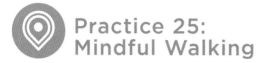

# Practice 25: Mindful Walking

Mindful walking is an ancient and effective practice for cultivating mindfulness. Take the time to experience this formal practice at least once. After that, if you'd like to continue with it, you can simply integrate it into your daily walking routine.

## TECHNIQUE

Choose a space for your practice where you can walk at least twelve steps before needing to turn. Open spaces such as beaches and fields are fabulous, but you can also practice in your own home. Remove your shoes, if possible. Practice for 5 to 10 minutes. Here's how:

1. Stand still and begin to settle your awareness into your body and onto your breath. Acknowledge to yourself that you are about to begin the practice of mindful walking.

2. Begin walking. Move with intent, but try not to change the way you're walking—just observe yourself.

3. Bring all of your attention to the sensations within your body:

- Start with your feet. Notice which part of your foot leaves the floor first, and which part touches it first. Notice how your toes respond to the motion of walking.

- Observe your ankle and knee joints. Watch how they extend, flex, and absorb impact.

- Become aware of the muscles in your thighs. Notice how they contract and flex as you move.

- Notice your hips and pelvis and how they move. Notice their multidirectional movements, and how they rotate and sway. Do these movements feel smooth or clunky to you?

- Explore the movements and sensations within your torso. Watch how your opposite hip and shoulder move in alignment through the gentle twist of your torso.

- Notice how your body feels as a whole. Does it feel heavy or light?

4. Turn your attention to your environment. Shift your awareness away from your body and toward the environment around you. Acknowledge what you see without analyzing it. Is your mind tempted to engage with the things you observe? If so, notice it and let it go.

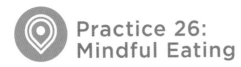

# Practice 26: Mindful Eating

Mindful eating is coming back into fashion. There's been a surge of interest in farm-to-table eating and in slow-cooked and home-cooked food—not to mention the ever-popular television cooking shows and the artful food photos that people love to share on social media. These days, it seems, we really want to be in touch with what we're eating. We want to appreciate our food visually, contemplate its origins, and nourish all of our senses through the act of eating, and that's a wonderful thing.

Practitioners of mindfulness have long known that paying attention to the act of eating is a powerful practice that can bring us into the present moment and change our experience in unexpected ways. Realistically, you probably wouldn't carry out the formal version of this practice every time you eat a meal, but it's a good idea to try it at least once; that way, you'll have planted the seed of mindful eating, and you'll be able to draw on it whenever you wish.

## TECHNIQUE

Choose a food you love, but haven't eaten recently (for this example we'll use a blueberry). It might be a piece of dark chocolate, a raisin, or a Brazil nut. Spend approximately 30 seconds at each stage of the instructions.

1. **Touching.** Hold the blueberry and explore it with your fingers and thumb. Feel its weight and texture. Approach it with a beginner's mind, as though it were the first time you'd ever held such a thing. You can even try holding the blueberry against your face to further explore its texture.

2. **Looking.** With beginner's eyes, look at the blueberry with curiosity. Take your time. With full awareness, explore every part of it; examine its color, its highlights, its shadows, grooves, and ridges.

3. **Smelling.** Now bring the blueberry to your nose and inhale. Explore its scent. Notice what happens within you. Is your mouth watering? Do any memories pop up? (If the food you are holding has no aroma, that's fine—simply notice that.)

### SPOTLIGHT ON SCIENCE

Research suggests that mindful eating might have therapeutic value for helping people with eating disorders—as well as improving healthy eating patterns in the general population—by enhancing awareness around hunger and satiety cues, improving one's sense of control around food, and diminishing depressive symptoms that can trigger emotional eating.

4. **Placing.** Be mindful as you bring the blueberry to your mouth. Allow it to touch your lips and notice again its texture. Notice, also, how your body reacts. You might sense an urge to bite down on the blueberry right away, or you might notice an increase in the flow of saliva. Now place the blueberry onto your tongue and, without chewing it, explore it with your mouth and tongue.

5. **Chewing.** Take your first bite with full awareness. Notice not only the taste but also the way your mouth and body respond. Imagine that you are experiencing the taste of the blueberry for the very first time.

6. **Swallowing.** Before you swallow, explore your desire to do so. How does your body indicate to you that it wants to swallow? Explore that feeling. Use your full awareness to see whether you can follow the sensations of the blueberry as you swallow it. If more blueberry remains in your mouth, continue chewing and swallowing as described.

7. **Reflecting.** As every wine connoisseur knows, the experience of taste can change over a few moments, and it always lingers after the act of swallowing. Take a moment to explore the aftertaste of the blueberry. Do you feel the urge to reach for another? Notice that, too.

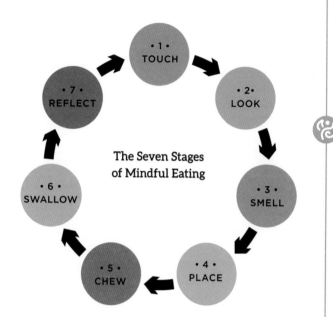

The Seven Stages of Mindful Eating

## ⬤ PRACTICE TIP

Now that you're familiar with the mindful eating practice, choose one mealtime each day and bring more mindful awareness to it. Do this on your own or share the experience with a friend or partner, or with your son or daughter. Children are great mindfulness practitioners and teachers, so why not invite them to explore this practice with you?

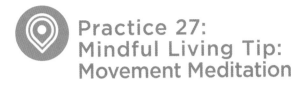

# Practice 27: Mindful Living Tip: Movement Meditation

Mindful movement meditations are definitely worth exploring. Some people find that they work really well, while others prefer less physical forms of meditative inquiry—but you might consider trying them before you rule them out. Yoga, for instance, is one of the most well-known forms of movement meditation that's practiced today (dance is another), but as with any and all of our activities, it may be practiced more or less mindfully, depending on the attitude and skill of the teacher and the student. These tips can help you infuse your next yoga session with even more mindful awareness.

1. **Begin and end with breath awareness.** Remain aware of your breath throughout your practice.

2. **Be gentle.** Stretch without striving; don't push yourself beyond your own personal limits. Bring an attitude of awareness, acceptance, and nonjudgment to your practice.

3. **Explore edges.** At the "soft edge" of a stretch, your body will tell you that something interesting is happening: You're exploring your body with a healthy intensity. At the "hard edge," the body has reached its current limit. Listen to these cues as they arise.

4. **Let the breath guide you.** The breath is the best gauge of the nervous system. It will tell you when you're approaching a "hard edge." Ease back a little, and let your breath guide you back to your "soft edge."

5. **Watch and allow.** When you mindfully explore the body, a wide range of physical and emotional sensations can arise. They can run the gamut from pleasant to unpleasant, but your approach to each should be the same: openness and acceptance. Let these sensations appear and let them go, without blocking them. Blocking sensations and emotions reinforces the tendency to avoid discomfort. But when you allow and accept them as they are, you're showing compassion toward yourself—and you're giving yourself the power to remain calm in the present moment, no matter how challenging that moment may be.

## Practice 28: Mindful Living Tip: Twenty Things

When do you feel most natural and in sync with yourself? What are the things you love to do so much that you lose track of time when you're doing them? Are you doing these things daily? Weekly? How many of them—if any—have you done this year?

Now that you've explored small, simple, daily joy rides (see Practice 24), it's time to widen your vision and explore the other activities and experiences that bring you the greatest joy.

### STEP 1

Create two columns with twenty lines in each. In the first column, list twenty things that you enjoy, once enjoyed, or even think you'll probably enjoy. Allow yourself to think beyond the things that you typically get to do, or could do, on a daily basis. For example, having a cup of tea is quite achievable on a daily basis, but the following activities are more likely to happen on a weekly, monthly, or annual basis: baking a cake for a friend, hiking, wandering around art galleries, traveling overseas, exploring a new city or suburb, camping, or soaking in the bath.

In the second column, write down the last time you engaged in each activity. It might have been two weeks, two years, or even two decades since you last revisited these pleasures—and that's perfectly fine.

### STEP 2

Now it's time to get out your calendar. Make time to experience at least one of these pleasures each month, and write it down so you won't forget. Keep your list somewhere handy so you can reflect on it from time to time.

---

### JOY MATTERS

The *Talmud*, an important Jewish text, advises that we will be called upon to account for all of the permitted pleasures in life that we neglected during our time on Earth.

---

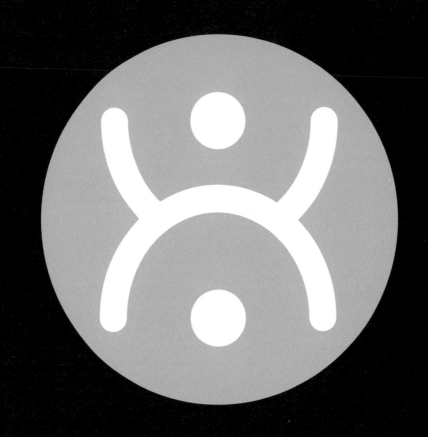

:: CHAPTER 7 ::

# TOUCHING PAIN

MEDITATION DOESN'T ACTUALLY FIX THE UNSETTLING REALITIES OF LIFE. IT CAN'T ALTER THE FACT THAT OUR MINDS WANDER. IT'S NOT A CURE FOR THE UNPLEASANT EMOTIONS THAT SURFACE, FROM TIME TO TIME, IN EACH OF US, AND IT CERTAINLY CAN'T WHISK US AWAY FROM THE REALITY OF PAIN AND SUFFERING. WHAT IT CAN DO IS HELP US CHANGE OUR RELATIONSHIP TO THESE THINGS, SO THAT THEY HAVE LESS IMPACT ON US.

The core principles and practices of mindfulness and meditation have been used for centuries to help people cope with the realities of living in a physical body that ages, gets sick, breaks down, and eventually dies. Modern science is playing catch-up, though, and it's only starting to investigate the practical processes by which these techniques help us better manage physical pain. Research shows that meditation and mindfulness are highly effective practices for managing pain, and they can improve coping and functional outcomes, reduce distress, and increase pain tolerance.

Studies suggest that meditation practices can help ease pain in two key ways: it can alter the brain's pain networks and can also reduce the stress, anxiety, and depression that often accompany (and even exacerbate) pain. Moreover, several studies indicate that open awareness styles of meditation (see chapter 4) are more effective than others for the specific management of pain.

### SPOTLIGHT ON SCIENCE

The application of mindfulness to pain management in the West began in the late 1970s with Dr. Jon Kabat-Zinn's stress reduction clinic at the University of Massachusetts, and it remains one of the best-researched fields of meditation.

Have you ever heard the saying "Pain is inevitable, but suffering is optional?" There's a great deal of truth to it. The primary experience of some pain is an unavoidable part of human existence. There is very little we can do about it except accept it, take steps to mitigate it, and move on. However, the secondary suffering we inflict upon ourselves by responding to our pain with anger, despair, judgment, and anxiety is something we *can* change. Mindfulness and meditation can help us distinguish between primary and secondary pain.

One form of primary pain that we all experience is the pain that arises in our physical bodies due to an injury or illness. This is the kind of pain you'll learn to work with in this chapter. It's unpleasant, and it's also inevitable. Secondary pain is, essentially, the mind's reaction to primary pain. Pain triggers negative feelings, which can drive negative thoughts; these, in turn, produce more negative feelings, and the result is a vicious cycle. Our negative thoughts about pain are often catastrophic and actually aggravate our relationship to the experience of pain, causing us to see it through a kind of tunnel vision. In situations like these, we can break that harmful cycle by getting some distance from our negative thoughts—by viewing them as mental events, and by staying with what's actually happening rather than getting lost in all of the negative mental chatter surrounding our experience.

Mindfulness training contradicts our natural (and understandable) approaches to pain, which range from ignoring or avoiding it to trying desperately to make it go away. Counterintuitively, mindfulness guides us to pay attention to pain with curiosity and nonjudgment.

Acceptance is also key. When we're experiencing pain, it's easy to get locked into a battle with it, and to insist that it shouldn't be happening. Yes, it's logical to want the suffering to stop, but the truth is that fighting with reality only creates additional suffering.

## ❶ KEY CONCEPT: ACCEPTANCE

Much of our suffering is caused when we refuse to accept life as it is. The situation we're refusing to accept could be an external event, such as a dog barking during our meditation practice, or it could be an internal experience, such as an unpleasant sensation, physical pain, a bad memory, or a distressing thought. Regardless of the nature of the experience, the bottom line is that life isn't the way we wanted it to be—and, like a cranky toddler, we refuse to accept that. We might rant and rave, or rush off in search of a source of pleasure to make us feel better. We avoid, reject, and "numb out" from anything that isn't exactly what we want. Then we chase after things we *do* want—even if those things aren't good for us in the short or long term. That's where mindfulness comes in. It transforms this madness into something much more manageable, and it cultivates our capacity for acceptance.

Acceptance is often a thorny concept for Westerners. They worry that "acceptance" might mean that they have to put up with unacceptable situations. However, research suggests that, in practice, this is simply not true. For example, in an eight-week study that was published in 2013, researchers found that participants assigned to a meditation course were five times more likely to help others when surreptitiously tested in a real-life situation. They didn't simply accept unfairness or injustice when they saw it. On the contrary: they *did* something about it.

### SPOTLIGHT ON SCIENCE

Research suggests that meditation might promote prosocial behavior by enhancing activity in an area of the brain known as the insula. The insula is linked to our ability to empathize with others. Meditators demonstrate greater brain-tissue density in the insula, which might explain why they're better able to take on another person's perspective.

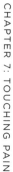

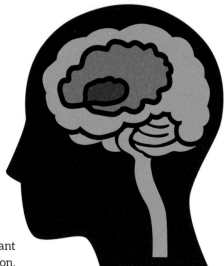

The insula (in red) is one important brain region activated by meditation.

## PRACTICES FOR WORKING WITH PAIN

If you've been working through the chapters in this book, you've already acquired some wonderful skills for working with pain. You've learned how to become aware of your own awareness, and how to direct it with intention, and you're able to both recognize and let go of judgment and analysis. Here are some additional tips for working specifically with pain when you're practicing some of the meditation techniques you've already encountered. Remember that all of the key concepts of nonjudgment, acceptance, and openness remain the same. Let your attitude toward pain mirror your attitude toward other physical sensations by neither chasing after it nor resisting it.

### BREATH

When you're using a breath-based practices (see chapter 3) to work with pain, continue to give priority to the breath. Let your breath take center stage, but allow your pain to be present backstage and in the wings. Note that it's there, and don't try to resist it. Then return your attention to the main event: your breath.

### BODY SCAN

The body scan meditation (see chapter 2) can be helpful for managing pain, because it gently draws your attention to individual parts of the body—and, inevitably, to the parts in which pain is present. The body scan meditation teaches you to be with your experience as it actually is: in an open and nonjudgmental way.

---

### PAIN MANAGEMENT TIP

There is no single right way to work with chronic pain, so it's important to develop your own tool kit of strategies. Your experience of pain is unique, so it makes sense that your repertoire of techniques for working with pain will be unique as well. It'll probably include one or more physical therapies, plus exercise, rest, and distraction. All of these can be effective when used appropriately. View meditation as another useful tool that's at your disposal. Try out the different techniques in this chapter—you've got nothing to lose by experimenting, right?—and adopt or adapt whatever works best for you.

---

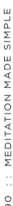

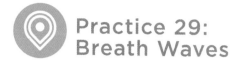

## Practice 29: Breath Waves

This practice combines breath awareness with another skill: learning to turn your awareness toward painful sensations in a gentle, open, and accepting way.

### TECHNIQUE

1. Find a position that's comfortable for you. If sitting is too painful, try standing or lying on your side (but do try to maintain a posture that's conducive to wakefulness).

2. Close your eyes and bring your awareness to your breath. Enjoy three full, slow, deep breaths. Fill the abdomen as you inhale and allow your entire body to soften as you exhale. Then allow your breath to settle into a natural rhythm.

3. Begin to ride the waves of each inhalation and exhalation. Focus on the tidal quality of the breath; notice how it ebbs and flows according to its own rhythm.

4. Now, turn your awareness toward an area of your body in which your feel pain, and direct your breath toward it.

5. As you inhale, draw the breath toward and into the area of sensation. As you exhale, let the breath depart from it.

6. Don't try to change the sensation of pain. Just draw your awareness to it, and feel the wave of your breath wash in and out.

7. You may notice that some of the pain sensations change over time as you continue to practice this technique—or you may not. It doesn't matter either way. The purpose of this practice isn't to change the sensations of pain, but to approach your pain in a different way.

8. When you're ready to complete your practice, return your awareness to your breath and enjoy three full, conscious breaths. Gently wiggle your fingers and toes. When you feel ready, slowly open your eyes.

### ⬤ PRACTICE TIP

Use this technique as needed. If you suffer from chronic pain, aim to practice this meditation for 10 to 20 minutes daily until you're familiar with it.

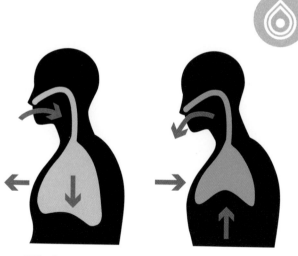

Ride the waves of your breath to open yourself
to your present experience.

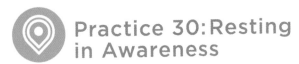

## Practice 30: Resting in Awareness

This practice adapts the skill of open awareness (see chapter 5) to apply specifically to pain.

### TECHNIQUE

1. Find a position that's comfortable for you. If sitting is too painful, try standing or lying on your side (but do try to maintain a posture that's conducive to wakefulness).

2. Close your eyes and bring your awareness to your breath. Enjoy three full, slow, deep breaths. Fill the abdomen as you inhale and allow your entire body to soften as you exhale. Then allow your breath to settle into a natural rhythm.

3. Now set your mind free. Let it roam and wander. It will soon become aware of something, perhaps a thought, sound, or physical sensation. Continue to let go of all of these as soon as they appear in your awareness, and become aware of the sense of awareness from which you have observed your own mind. Curiously notice this undercurrent of awareness.

4. Whenever your mind is distracted by the sensation of pain, pay attention to your awareness of that pain. Notice how your awareness of pain is not in pain, even though your body may be experiencing sensations of pain. This suggests that there are aspects of your being that are larger than your pain. Awareness is larger than pain. Your awareness is free, unencumbered, and unaffected by the experience of pain.

5. Practice noticing the awareness that notices the pain. In doing so, open yourself to the full spectrum of your life experience. Consciously let your awareness roam the myriad of non-pain-related sensations within you and around you. Direct your awareness to the spaces between things (revisit Practice 21 in chapter 5). Your experience is far more expansive than the limited experience of pain.

6. When you're ready to complete your practice, return your awareness to your breath and enjoy three full, conscious breaths. Gently wiggle your fingers and toes. When you feel ready, slowly open your eyes.

### ⬤ PRACTICE TIP

Use this technique as needed. If you suffer from chronic pain, aim to practice this meditation for 10 to 20 minutes daily until you're familiar with it.

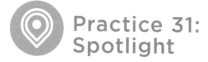

# Practice 31: Spotlight

In this exercise, you'll learn to use the sensations of pain as the anchor for your awareness. This practice may seem counterintuitive, since it guides your meditative awareness toward the pain itself, but the act of staying with the experience of pain can be transformative; it can help us break the habitual and unhelpful patterns of pain avoidance in which we try to ignore or deny the experience of the present moment—causing us to suffer more, not less.

## TECHNIQUE

1. Find a position that's comfortable for you. If sitting is too painful, try standing or lying on your side (but do try to maintain a posture that's conducive to wakefulness).

2. Close your eyes and bring your awareness to your breath. Enjoy three full, slow, deep breaths. Fill the abdomen as you inhale and allow your entire body to soften as you exhale. Then allow your breath to settle into a natural rhythm.

3. As you simply watch your breath, call upon the key concepts of acceptance, openness, curiosity, and nonjudgment. You might like to refamiliarize yourself with these concepts and briefly contemplate what they mean to you. Apply these attitudes to the act of breath awareness.

4. Now direct your attention to an area of your body in which you feel pain. Try not to push the pain away. Instead, use these sensations as a way to connect with the experience of the present moment.

5. Begin to explore the painful sensations. (This is not an invitation to *think* about them, but to *feel* them. If thoughts or emotions arise, simply see them for what they are—mind stuff—and redirect your awareness back to the sensations of pain.) Because of our natural tendency to avoid pain or to distract ourselves from it, this might sound a little scary. If that's true for you, take a moment to contemplate that you already have pain (and if you suffer from chronic pain, you may have had it for a long time). So you have nothing to lose by trying a new approach to working with it.

6. Now dive more deeply into the area of painful sensations. Feel into the sensation, and explore the edge of where the pain begins to dissipate and where it intensifies. Stay with your experience, whatever it is. Notice whether the pain is static and still, or moving and changing. Lay out the welcome mat for whatever's currently present in your experience (you might as well: it's already here, anyway!).

7. Move into the center of the pain. Again, with great curiosity, feel what arises within that center. Observe it. Does it have a temperature? Is it moving or static? Is it dense or diffuse? Solid or loose? Once again, this is not an invitation to *think* about the painful sensation, but to *feel* it. Without judgment, explore the specific sensations that comprise the totality of pain.

8. Now, draw your awareness back a bit from the center of the painful sensation, and extend it again to include the entire area of pain. Have any of the sensations changed? It doesn't matter either way. The purpose of this practice isn't to change the sensations of pain, but to approach your pain in a different way.

9. You might wish to repeat steps 5 to 8 a couple of times, turning the spotlight of your awareness toward and close to the painful sensations, then pulling back a little.

10. Extend your awareness to the rest of your body and notice other sensations there. If you find more than one area of pain, you can repeat the process for each area. If not, simply direct your awareness—along with your attitude of acceptance, curiosity, and nonjudgment—into different areas of your body, part by part.

11. When you're ready to complete your practice, return your awareness to your breath and enjoy three full, conscious breaths. Gently wiggle your fingers and toes. When you feel ready, slowly open your eyes.

## ○ PRACTICE TIP

Use this technique as needed. If you suffer from chronic pain, aim to practice this meditation for 10 to 20 minutes daily until you're familiar with it.

### SPOTLIGHT ON SCIENCE

Participants taught mindful breathing techniques for only 20 minutes over a 3-day period were tested to see how reactive they were to mild and stronger electrical shocks. After the mindfulness training, the participants experienced significantly less anxiety, less suffering from pain, and less reactivity to the pain relative to where they were beforehand.

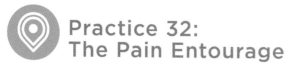

# Practice 32:
# The Pain Entourage

In this technique, you'll learn to bring your attention to the thoughts and feelings—also known as the pain entourage—that often accompany (and frequently worsen) the experience of pain.

## TECHNIQUE

1. Find a position that's comfortable for you. If sitting is too painful, try standing or lying on your side (but do try to maintain a posture that's conducive to wakefulness).

2. Close your eyes and bring your awareness to your breath. Enjoy three full, slow, deep breaths. Fill the abdomen as you inhale and allow your entire body to soften as you exhale. Then allow your breath to settle into a natural rhythm.

3. Guide your awareness to, and focus on, the painful sensations in your body. Try to stay with these sensations with openness and acceptance. If this becomes too difficult, return your awareness to your breath.

4. As you rest your awareness on the sensations of pain, it's likely that you'll soon be distracted by thoughts and emotions. In meditation, we usually notice and let go of any thoughts and feelings that arise, but in this pain-specific practice, we'll turn directly toward them. So, be alert to the thoughts and feelings that arise in connection with the painful sensations, and pay particular attention to them.

5. Explore your thoughts about pain. Notice that even the word *pain* is a thought. It is one way of describing what's happening. But in its barest form, what's happening in your body is a sensation. What happens when you apply the word *sensation* to your experience, instead of *pain*?

6. Notice any other thoughts that come up in connection with pain. Perhaps you're thinking, "This is unbearable," or "Will this ever go away?" or "I can't live like this." Just for a moment, consider that none of these thoughts is actually the experience of pain itself. They are thoughts about pain. See them for what they are: thoughts about pain, not the experience of pain itself. Approach them as if they were thought-clouds drifting by on the wide-open sky of your awareness.

7. Observe your emotions about pain in the same way. You might be experiencing irritability, anger, frustration, sadness, or despair. Remember that these are emotions, not the sensation of pain itself. For a moment, just watch these emotions as emotions, and let them be.

8. Now drop the storyline of these thoughts and emotions. Allow your awareness to extend beyond your thoughts and emotions about the painful sensations (though these thoughts and emotions may still be present in the background), and shift your attention toward the painful sensations themselves. Notice only the pain, minus the entourage of pain-related thoughts and feelings. Explore bare sensation itself.

9. Extend your awareness even further. Let your experience of the sensation of pain join the thoughts and feelings about pain that are lingering in the background, and allow your awareness to roam into whatever else is happening for you in the present moment: you may be experiencing other sensations, other emotions, or things happening in your external environment.

10. As you let your awareness roam free, notice how expansive your awareness really is. Observe the way in which it is separate from the objects it perceives. Notice how your awareness of pain is not *in* pain, even though your body may be experiencing sensations of pain. This suggests that there are aspects of your being that are larger than your pain. Awareness is larger than pain. Your awareness is free, unencumbered, and unaffected by the experience of pain.

11. When you're ready to complete your practice, return your awareness to your breath and enjoy three full, conscious breaths. Gently wiggle your fingers and toes. When you feel ready, slowly open your eyes.

## ◌ PRACTICE TIP

Use this technique as needed. If you suffer from chronic pain, aim to practice this meditation for 10 to 20 minutes daily until you're familiar with it.

# Practice 33: Mindful Living Tip: Wise Waiting

Many of life's moments take place in the "waiting spaces" between things: between appointments, during commutes, waiting for the taxi, waiting for the kettle to boil, and while standing in line at the store. We wait for pages to load and for movies to download; we wait for babies to fall asleep and for partners to wake up, and in the midst of much of this waiting, our minds (and sometimes our bodies) wander. Sometimes, we try to cram something into the empty space. Other times, we watch the seconds tick by as we tap our feet and sigh. Or we grab our phones, distracting ourselves with technology. Few of us stay present to what is; few of us are immersed in the moment, at peace with waiting, and even delightedly curious to discover more about what the moment holds—even though we know that such mindfulness enhances our happiness.

By now, you already have all the tools you need to practice wise waiting in moments like these. This exercise is merely an invitation to apply those skills to those moments—when you're standing in a long line or in front of a kettle that still hasn't boiled.

## STEP 1

Set your intention to cultivate mindfulness by picking one or two waiting spaces that happen regularly in your life (like waiting for the bus, or for your son to wake up from his nap). Take a moment to reflect on your habits. What have you been doing during this waiting period?

## STEP 2

Review, choose, and apply your tools. You have dozens of mindfulness techniques to use in these moments. Consider different breathing practices (chapter 1), or explore your sensory experience (chapter 2). You might settle into a body scan (chapter 2), immerse yourself in mantra meditation or breath meditation (chapter 3), watch your own mind (chapter 4), or expand your awareness to notice the space within and around you (chapter 5).

Then watch how present-moment awareness infuses your life with a greater sense of calm, clarity, and connectedness.

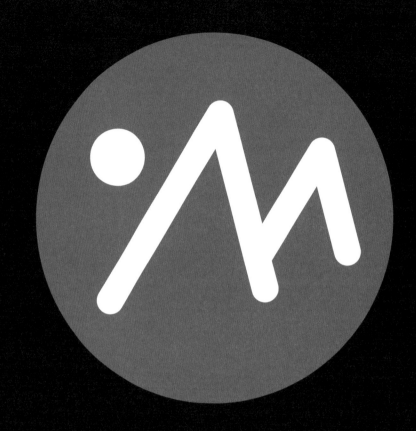

## CHAPTER 8

# ENCOUNTERING DIFFICULT EMOTIONS

IT'S RELATIVELY EASY TO OBSERVE OURSELVES, AND EVEN TO LOVE OURSELVES, WHEN WE LIKE WHAT WE SEE. AND IT'S NOT USUALLY DIFFICULT TO STAY WITH OUR OWN EMOTIONS WHEN THEY ARE JOYFUL, CONFIDENT, KIND, AND LOVING. BUT IT'S HARDER TO STAY PRESENT WITH OURSELVES WHEN WE DON'T LIKE WHAT WE SEE. WE TYPICALLY RESPOND BY TURNING AWAY WHEN WE ENCOUNTER EMOTIONS THAT ARE UNPLEASANT OR FRIGHTENING—AND WE END UP STUCK IN OUR CYCLICAL PATTERNS OF HABITUAL REACTIVITY AND AVOIDANCE.

Yes, when it comes to encountering unpleasant emotions, many of us react out of habit. We might respond with irritability, with procrastination and avoidance, or with overeating, overworking, or other addictive behaviors that can help us numb out and avoid the reality of our unsettling emotions. Some of us even lash out at others with hurtful, unhelpful words we'll later regret, simply because we haven't been able to face our own emotional states quietly and mindfully. Others retreat into themselves and enter a cave of self-defeat and depression. We each have a unique pattern when it comes to responding, avoiding, and denying our own difficult emotions—and it rarely results in overcoming them and living mindfully.

Meditation and mindfulness teach us that we don't need to avoid or repress any part of our life experiences. No matter how painful, unpleasant, distressing, or frightening an experience is, we can rest assured that we can hold it within the spaciousness of our awareness—and our awareness itself is never affected in any way. Like the sky on a stormy day, awareness restfully watches the crackle and crash of lightning and thunder, it doesn't become them. It isn't tainted by them. It simply accepts the current situation as it is, and wisely waits for the storm to pass.

The tools of meditation allow us to look more closely at our life experiences. They teach us acceptance, nonjudgment, curiosity, and how to remain in the present moment. They show us that our awareness is far more expansive than we ever thought possible, and they guide us to befriend all parts of ourselves with great compassion.

Meditation and mindfulness give us the skills to observe the rising and passing of our emotions. The wisdom that all things are transient becomes our own inner experience, not just a bumper-sticker platitude.

If we don't understand the principles of meditation, turning to face our emotional suffering could easily make things appear worse than they actually are. We imagine it could be truly terrifying to face up to the extent of our craziness, rage, criticism, jealousy, or insecurity, but the meditative approach isn't harsh. The whole purpose is to loosen the delusionary aspects of our minds, and the process is, in fact, a gentle one.

This chapter will guide you toward emotional suffering. You'll be asked to put aside your usual way of reacting when you encounter negative feelings. This might be a challenge for the fixers and problem-solvers among us, but it's also an invitation to experiment with a new and powerful strategy for coping with everyday life. Problems can often be solved—but emotions? Not so much. Sometimes, emotions can only be felt, and to feel them means to acknowledge them, inhabit them, and let go of the habitual drive to "fix" or "solve" them. All we need to do is to acknowledge and accept their presence. Often, this is the gentle touch that can help them change of their own accord, but that's not why we're here. We're not setting out to alter or mask our difficult emotions. We're here to experience them, to experience life, to taste all that's on offer—and to dance with both the darkness and the light.

# ❶ KEY CONCEPT: HOSPITALITY

As mindful meditators, we survive and even thrive on negative emotions by cultivating an attitude of hospitality toward them. This means that we welcome everything, resist nothing, accommodate graciously, and let go gracefully.

As gracious hosts of our emotions, we must attend to each and every visitor. We don't turn anyone away at the door. We keep them all in perspective, accepting each visitor without becoming overly invested in any of them..

One way to apply this hospitality to unpleasant emotions is to recognize them by literally greeting them when you become aware of their presence. You might say aloud, or silently to yourself, "Oh, hello, insecurity. You're here again," or "Hi there, boredom. It's you."

This practice of greeting brings our awareness into the present moment. It lends us a degree of space, which helps us avoid being caught up in an emotional storm. It awakens the witness, and in that brief moment, we are both experiencing *and* witnessing ourselves experiencing the emotion. Greeting an emotion in this way can also serve as a reminder that, like all visitors, this guest isn't here to stay. It'll soon pack its suitcase and will be on its way.

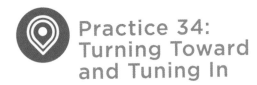

## Practice 34: Turning Toward and Tuning In

This practice uses a difficult emotion as an anchor for being in the present moment. It guides you to stay with uncomfortable emotions, and supports you in exploring them intimately by focusing on the way in which they manifest in your body. You'll need to bring a challenging emotion to mind, and it's best to start with something lightweight. Don't begin with the serious, heavy aftereffects of a major trauma. Focus instead on a mild experience of irritation, sadness, or any other emotion you wish to work with.

### TECHNIQUE

1. Set aside some time during which you can be alone and undisturbed. Sit in any position that's comfortable for you, and close your eyes.

2. Begin by gently moving your attention to the process of breathing. Enjoy three full, slow, deep breaths. Fill your abdomen as you inhale, and allow your entire body to soften as you exhale. Then allow your breath to settle into a natural rhythm.

3. Bring your awareness to your senses, and spend 10 to 30 seconds on each sense. Explore sound, smell, taste, touch, and vision.

4. Bring an unpleasant emotion to mind. Allow it to take center stage in your awareness.

5. Shift your awareness to discover how this feeling manifests in your body. If you can, find physical signs of the emotion in several parts of your body—such as heat in your face or tightness in your chest due to anger, or a sense of heaviness in your stomach due to sadness—then move your attention to the area in which they're strongest.

6. Direct your breath to this area, allowing each inhalation to wash in and out. Turn toward and tune in to the sensation. Does it have a temperature? Is it moving or static? Dense or diffuse? This is not an invitation to *think* about the sensation, but to *feel* it without judgment. Remember that you're not trying to change your experience; you're simply staying with your experience as it is. If you like, say to yourself, "It's okay to feel this emotion."

7. Notice whether any resistance to staying with your experience arises. Do you feel the urge to fix it or avoid it? Notice this, too, and see if you can apply mindfulness to this experience as well by bringing an openhearted curiosity to the resistance itself.

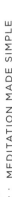

**8.** Notice whether a storyline about the emotion appears. If so, that's okay. Just notice these thoughts for what they are— thoughts. Let go of the storyline and keep returning your awareness to the area of your body in which the emotion is physically strongest. Again, this is not an invitation to *think* about the sensations, but to *feel* them. Turn toward them with loving acceptance.

**9.** Stay with the bodily sensations of the emotion. Let them be. Accept them. Soften up to them. Say a silent "yes" to them, signifying that you're allowing them to be just as they are. Another way to allow them space is to imagine the edges of the sensation softening and merging or blending with your entire body. Allow them to be present. Allow them to take up space in your body and being. Embrace them with loving acceptance, and notice what happens— without judgment—when you do this.

**10.** If you wish, you can repeat steps 4 to 9, focusing on another area of the body that holds the sensations associated with the emotion.

**11.** When you're ready to complete your practice, return your awareness to your breath and enjoy three full, conscious breaths. Gently wiggle your fingers and toes. When you feel ready, slowly open your eyes, and bring your awareness to the space you're in.

##  PRACTICE TIPS

Aim to practice this meditation for 10 to 20 minutes daily. You can use a mini version of this practice whenever you find yourself in the midst of an unsettling emotion. This will quickly give you some distance from (and curiosity about) how the emotion is making itself felt. Even a small amount of distance from the emotion can help break habitual reaction patterns.

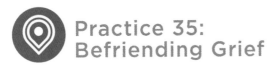

## Practice 35: Befriending Grief

Grief can be exhausting. We might feel depleted, defeated, and deflated by our loss, and sometimes we aren't sure how to go on.

Meditation can provide our tired, grieving hearts and minds with respite. It can replenish our nervous systems, and it can help us be present with ourselves; remaining present with grief facilitates healing. We do this gently, because connecting with grief means touching a place of great tenderness within the self. In this way, grief can be a pathway to profound compassion. So, hold yourself and your grief as if you were cradling a vulnerable child. As you hold that space, know that it is larger than the experience itself. You are larger than this grief, and in the spaciousness of your awareness, you are able to host this grief and heal from it. Remember, however strong your grief may be, it is also entirely ordinary. It's an integral part of being human.

### TECHNIQUE

1. Set aside some time during which you can be alone and undisturbed. Sit in any position that's comfortable for you, and close your eyes.

2. Begin by gently moving your attention to the process of breathing. Enjoy three full, slow, deep breaths. Fill your abdomen as you inhale, and allow your entire body to soften as you exhale. Then allow your breath to settle into a natural rhythm.

3. Rest your awareness on the anchor of your breath (or choose another anchor, such as a mantra), and notice that your mind will soon be tugged by distractions, sensations, thoughts, and feelings.

4. When the feeling of grief arises, allow it to take center stage in your awareness. For this meditation, give yourself permission to leave the anchor of your breath—knowing that you can come back to it at any moment—and allow your mind to wander to any aspect of your grief.

#### SPOTLIGHT ON SCIENCE

Studies of women with cancer suggest that mindfulness can assist with the processes of grief and psychological adjustment to a cancer diagnosis. In other research, promising findings indicate that mindfulness may significantly reduce the incidence of ongoing depression in bereaved elderly following the loss of a loved-one.

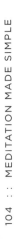

5. Label the aspects of grief that arise in your mind as "remembering," "reminiscing," "worrying," "anger," or whatever else comes up for you. All of these manifestations are facets of your grief. Allow them to be present, and let them wash in and out of your awareness.

6. Now, watch the part of you that's watching these experiences within your own mind. Become aware of awareness itself, and ask yourself whether this aware part of you actually dwells *in* grief. You'll probably discover that the answer is no, even though you're in the midst of the emotion. This suggests that there are aspects of your being that are larger than your suffering and your grief. Awareness is larger than grief.

7. Allow your awareness to gently hold the space in which your grief is present. Cradle both yourself and the emotion in the loving embrace of your all-encompassing, compassionate awareness. Accept whatever arises. It's okay if you start to cry, for example; allow it to happen and keep on cradling yourself and this grief. If the crying or sobbing becomes too intense, you can pause and take a few moments to focus on long, slow breathing before you continue.

8. When you're ready to complete your practice, return your awareness to your breath and enjoy three full, conscious breaths. Gently wiggle your fingers and toes. Become aware of the space around you before you slowly open your eyes.

## ⬤ PRACTICE TIP
Aim to practice this meditation for 10 to 20 minutes as needed. You can revisit this practice at different times, even if it didn't resonate with you the first time you tried it.

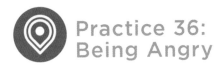

## Practice 36: Being Angry

Anger is an easier emotion to explore through meditation because it's generally associated with very strong physical sensations, which can act as a way to connect to the present moment. However, people often hope to avoid their anger, believing that it is inherently "bad," or that it reflects a character flaw. Let's get one thing straight: anger is just one of myriad human emotions, and, like all mind states, it can be handled more or less consciously. As mindfulness meditators, we choose to move in the direction of bringing greater consciousness to all of our experiences. When the anger's energy is harnessed productively, it can be used to make positive changes to our own situations and to the world around us. When it's mismanaged, it can be the most destructive forces on the planet.

### TECHNIQUE

1. Sit in any position that's comfortable for you and close your eyes.

2. Move your attention to the process of breathing. Fill your abdomen as you inhale and allow your entire body to soften as you exhale, then let your breath settle into a natural rhythm. Let the breath breathe you.

3. Now scan your body from your head to your feet, and, with curiosity, discover where you can feel the physical sensations associated with the emotion of anger. Anger is often experienced as a sense of heat or tightness in the stomach or the muscles in the neck, jaws, and shoulders. Explore your experience with openness and curiosity. (If you aren't currently experiencing anger but still wish to try this practice, bring to mind a recent situation in which you felt angry. Imagine the situation in detail and allow yourself to let the feeling of anger surface again.)

4. Direct your attention to the physical sensation in your body that's the most associated with anger. Begin to explore the sensation. Become intimate with it. This is not an invitation to *think* about the sensation, but to *feel* it. If thoughts or emotions arise, simply see them for what they are—mind stuff—and then redirect your awareness back to the sensation. Feeling into the sensation, explore the edge of where it begins to dissipate and where it intensifies. Stay with your experience, whatever it is. Notice whether the sensation is static or moving. Lay out the welcome mat for whatever is currently present in your experience (you might as well: it's already here, anyway!).

5. Now move into the center of the sensation. Again, with great curiosity, feel what arises there. Does it have a temperature? Is it moving or static? Is it dense or diffuse? Solid or loose? Once again, this is not an invitation to *think* about the sensation, but to *feel* it without judgment.

6. It's likely that you'll be distracted by thoughts and emotions. Try to stay open to the fact that anxious or angry thoughts have arisen. Let them come and go in the background as you maintain your awareness of the physical sensations in the foreground.

7. Now, draw your awareness back a little from the center of the sensation, and focus on it as a whole. Has the sensation changed during the time you've been noticing it? It doesn't matter either way; the purpose of this practice isn't to change the sensation, but to approach it in a different way.

8. You might wish to repeat steps 4 to 7, shining the spotlight of your awareness on the physical sensations associated with anger. Hover up close to the sensation, then draw back a little.

9. Extend your awareness and notice other sensations in your body. As always, do so with an attitude of acceptance, curiosity, and nonjudgment. Explore your body, part by part: feet, legs, torso, arms, hands, and head.

10. Now become aware of the part of you that's watching these experiences within your own mind. Become aware of awareness itself.

11. When you're ready to complete your practice, return your awareness to your breath and enjoy three full, conscious breaths. Gently wiggle your fingers and toes. Become aware of the space around you before you slowly open your eyes.

##  PRACTICE TIP

Aim to practice this meditation for 10 to 20 minutes. Use as needed.

### SPOTLIGHT ON SCIENCE

Mindfulness could be a useful treatment for addressing aggression. Research has shown that it can counteract factors associated with anger, such as rumination, low self-regulation, lack of present-moment awareness, and low empathy.

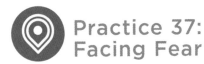 ## Practice 37: Facing Fear

Realizing that fear is a mind state and isn't necessarily based upon fact allows us to respond to it more consciously. Meditation helps us develop the metacognitive awareness in which we are better able to see anxious thoughts for what they are—just thoughts. Meditation also teaches us that we can choose where to place our attention, and it gives us the confidence to face our emotions directly because we know that we're far more spacious than these transitory states. We soon realize that we can direct our awareness toward fear, or away from it.

## TECHNIQUE

1. Sit in any position that's comfortable for you, and close your eyes.

2. Begin by gently moving your attention to the process of breathing. Enjoy three full, slow, deep breaths. Fill your abdomen as you inhale and allow your entire body to soften as you exhale. Then let your breath settle into a natural rhythm.

3. Spend several moments simply resting your awareness on your breath. Become aware that you are breathing without making a conscious effort to change your breathing patterns.

4. Now, take a moment to name what you're feeling. Know that the emotion state you're

### SPOTLIGHT ON SCIENCE

Compelling research from cognitive neuroscientists indicates that meditation changes brain structures and functions in ways that help decrease and manage fear and anxiety. Specifically, mindfulness meditation has been found to *decrease* activity and brain cell volume in the amygdala, which is a key player in generating fear, anxiety, and stress.

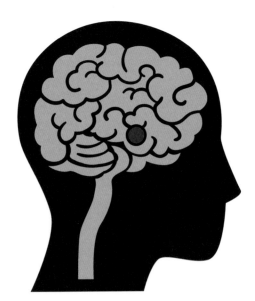

The amygdala (in red) activates the fear response.

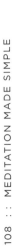

experiencing is fear (or you might use another name, such as anxiety). Recognize the emotion for what it is. (If you're not currently experiencing fear but wish to try this practice, imagine in detail a recent situation in which you felt fearful and allow yourself to let the fear surface again.)

5. Notice the physical sensations associated with fear. Perhaps your heart is pumping or your chest feels tight. You might be clenching your fists, sweating, or shaking. Notice these sensations with a curious and open attitude. Be interested in what you find. Continue to scan your body for signs of fear and stress.

6. Now seek out the area in your body where the sensations are most intense and turn toward it. Lean into it and explore what you find there. Approach it with an attitude of compassion, and direct your breath to it. As you inhale, draw your breath toward and into the sensations. As you exhale, let the breath depart from the area. Don't try to change the sensation of fear; draw your awareness to it, and feel your breath wash in and out.

7. You may begin to notice that some of the sensations change over time as you continue to breathe, or you may not. It doesn't matter either way. The purpose of this practice isn't to change the sensations of fear but to approach it in a different way.

8. It's likely that you'll be distracted by thoughts and emotions. Maintain an open and accepting attitude toward the fact that anxious thoughts have arisen. Let them

come and go in the background as you maintain your awareness of the physical sensations. Keep the physical sensations at the center of your awareness and allow thoughts to come and go, seeing them for what they are—just thoughts.

9. You might wish to repeat steps 5 to 8 again, focusing on another area in which the physical sensations associated with fear are present in your body.

10. Now, watch the part of you that's watching these experiences within your own mind. Become aware of awareness itself, and ask yourself whether this aware part of you actually dwells *in* fear. You'll probably discover that the answer is no, even though you're in the midst of fear. This suggests that there are aspects of your being that are larger than your fear. Awareness is larger than fear.

11. When you're ready to complete your practice, return your awareness to your breath and enjoy three full, conscious breaths. Gently wiggle your fingers and toes. Become aware of the space around you before you slowly open your eyes.

## ⬤ PRACTICE TIPS

Aim to practice this meditation for 10 to 20 minutes. Use as needed. If you struggle with anxiety and fear, then it's a good idea to become familiar with this meditation technique before you "need" it. Work with it during your formal practice by bringing to mind a time at which you felt anxious.

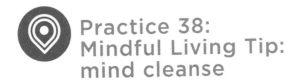

# Practice 38:
# Mindful Living Tip:
# mind cleanse

We live in a world that's jam packed with technology. In fact, according to a report by the UN, more people have mobile phones than access to clean water. Thanks to technological advances, the amount of information to which we're exposed—and the number of media sources that are clamoring for our attention—has grown exponentially. This isn't an exaggeration: researchers have calculated that between the internet, 24-hour television, and mobile phones, we now receive five times as much information per day than we did in 1986, and yet we're working with the same brains. In fact, we're working with the same brains with which our ancestors wandered the savannah, and these brains can easily become overstimulated and addicted to consuming information.

Giving up technology altogether isn't the solution. We simply need to learn to give our brains a break and to make conscious, mindful choices about what we allow them to consume. Our appetites for technology are best managed in the same way that we manage our appetites for food—mindfully, and, as psychotherapist Carl Jung remarked, with some degree of self-control.

This mind cleanse practice is just like a food cleanse. It simply asks us to pay attention to what we're consuming so that we can establish a baseline, and then we'll develop and execute a conscious plan to consume a smaller amount of higher-quality information.

## STEP 1

Take a moment to explore how you currently feed your mind with technology. How many hours of television do you watch each day or each week? How much time do you spend surfing online and reading or writing emails? What about social media? Keep an honest record and you'll discover how much time you really spend scrolling through the lives of others and curating your own life to present to the world.

## STEP 2

Make a goal and set a plan. Do you want to do a "cold turkey" cleanse? This may be difficult for many people, since computers, email, and even social media outlets are part of their work lives. If that sounds like you, try limiting your email check-in times (for example, restrict yourself to morning, lunchtime, and late afternoon). Or confine your social media use to 10 minutes per day.

Perhaps you want your cleanse to focus on the quality as well as the quantity of what you're feeding your mind. Which television shows, websites, or social media sites do you consider worthwhile, and which add very little to your life?

Feeding your mind with high-quality "food" means letting go of the low-grade stuff. It's about moving beyond things that are no longer serving you. It requires mindful discernment (to tell the difference between low and high quality), assertiveness (to say no to what doesn't make the cut), and courage (to move ahead with your choices). When we're on the path of mindfulness, we often find that we already instinctively know what serves us and what doesn't. It's just that we've gotten a bit muddled, and aren't paying close attention to the subtle signs in our bodies and minds that can help us make the healthiest choices.

Think about the length of your cleanse; I recommend trying it for 2 weeks. At the end of the trial period, you might decide you want to keep it up, or you might want to change your habits in other ways. You might even wish to return to your precleanse habits. It's up to you.

## STEP 3

Get underway and seek support. You might find that it's helpful to let other people know what you're doing and, if necessary, to seek their support. As with any cleanse, be prepared for some withdrawal symptoms and cravings. These signals are valuable in themselves: by showing us just how addicted to technology we've become.

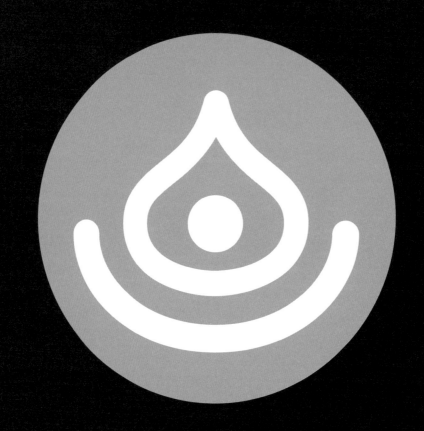

:: CHAPTER 9 ::

# EQUANIMITY IN CHALLENGING TIMES

ALL OF LIFE IS MEDICINE, AS THE SAYING GOES. IN OTHER WORDS, ALL OF OUR EXPERIENCES CAN HELP US GROW AND HEAL THE PARTS OF OURSELVES THAT MIGHT FEEL ROUGH AND JAGGED. CHALLENGING TIMES ARE THE PERFECT TESTING GROUNDS FOR MINDFULNESS PRACTICES. THEY ALLOW US TO EXPLORE OUR EDGES AND APPLY OUR SKILLS WHERE THEY MATTER MOST: OUR DAILY LIVES.

It's relatively easy to be present and accepting when everything is going according to plan, but the difficult moments truly test our balance. In this chapter, you'll learn a helpful mindfulness technique used by cognitive behavioral therapists for specifically applying mindfulness to life's trickier areas—the places where our balance falters a little bit.

## ❶ KEY CONCEPT: EQUANIMITY

**Equanimity** is a term that's rarely encountered outside of meditation circles, yet it's one of the most beautiful and important concepts for mindfulness practitioners. It means "even mind," or the ability to be calm, even, composed, balanced, level-headed, reasoned, and self-controlled, regardless of what's going on around us.

**Equanimity** derives from the Latin word *aequus*, meaning "balanced," and *animus*, meaning "spirit" or "internal state." It is defined as mental or emotional stability or composure, especially under tension or strain.

When we are equanimous, we accept the reality of our current situation. We accept whatever has arisen in either our internal or our external landscapes—but we don't get swept up and carried away by it. The Dalai Lama phrases it best: "With equanimity, you can deal with situations with calm and reason while keeping your inner happiness."

Equanimity applies equally to things we'd consider to be bad and things we'd consider to be good. When we act with equanimity, we respond with balance and composure, regardless of circumstances and events.

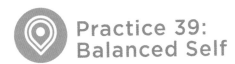

# Practice 39: Balanced Self

This technique is very similar to a method psychotherapists use to fuse mindfulness practices with traditional **cognitive behavioral therapy (CBT)**. Several therapeutic approaches offer this blend, and the technique you'll learn here is adapted from one that's taught in Mindfulness-integrated Cognitive Behavioral Therapy (MiCBT).

**Cognitive behavioral therapy (CBT)** teaches individuals to recognize and address unhelpful thought patterns, feelings, and behaviors. Both mindfulness and CBT can increase a person's awareness of negative thoughts and behaviors, although they're two different techniques. Mindfulness practices focus on noticing and accepting thoughts and feelings without reacting to them, while CBT tends to focus on challenging those thoughts and explicitly changing behavior patterns. Recent research suggests that a combination of these approaches, known as Mindfulness-based Cognitive Therapy or Mindfulness-integrated Cognitive Behavioral Therapy, is as effective as antidepressants for reducing relapse rates for recurrent depression.

To practice this technique, you'll use not only your mindfulness and meditation skills but also your ability to visualize. You'll be guided to bring to mind a challenging situation, and you'll be asked to contemplate both the worst-case and the best-case scenarios for it. Most important, you'll practice being equanimous—that is, balanced and composed—in your response, regardless of whether the outcome is positive or negative.

For instance, you might like to imagine an upcoming conversation you need to have with Angela, a coworker, about an error in her work. Your habitual pattern of interacting with Angela is something you'd like to work on. Perhaps you're typically very short with her, or are even rude to her, when—in your opinion—she tries to shirk her responsibilities. During the balanced self practice, you'll visualize the upcoming conversation you'll have with her. You'll begin by imagining the worst-case scenario for this conversation. In it, you might imagine that Angela insists that the error is not hers, and that she can't do anything to reduce the potential for future errors. As you visualize this worst-case scenario, you'll allow yourself to truly experience whatever arises in your body while remaining open, accepting, and equanimous toward these sensations. You'll also imagine yourself remaining calm and equanimous throughout the encounter. You'll call upon your mindfulness skills to help you remain present in the situation by feeling into your body and the space you're in. You'll bring a sense of openness and acceptance to the situation as it is—which, in this case, is obviously not as you would like it to be.

After 5 minutes of visualizing the worst-case scenario, you'll take a rest period in which you practice breath meditation (see Practice 9). Then you'll begin to imagine the best-case scenario for another 5 minutes, and again, you'll practice staying balanced, accepting, and composed.

This exercise teaches us about our desires and our attachment to making sure that events unfold in a certain way—our way. By practicing remaining balanced, regardless of the outcome, we cultivate the ability to be mindful in the real world rather than being tossed around by our desires, attachments, and disappointments. It helps us let go of our unrealistic expectations of how the world should be. That way, we can live more mindfully and artfully in the present moments of our lives as they actually are.

## TECHNIQUE

*NOTE: THIS TECHNIQUE SHOULD BE PRACTICED AT THE END OF A 10- TO 20-MINUTE MEDITATION SESSION.*

1. Choose an upcoming situation that's challenging for you. It's best to start with an irritating or mildly challenging situation rather than a traumatic or emotionally intense issue. Bring this situation to the front of your mind.

2. **5 Minutes: Worst-Case Scenario.** Visualize the worst-case scenario for this situation and simultaneously visualize yourself remaining equanimous throughout it. Allow yourself to experience any physical sensations that occur as you imagine this scenario. You might experience muscle tension (clenching your jaw, or neck and shoulder tension), increased heart rate, perspiration, or tightness in the chest. Let yourself move close to these sensations without trying to change them. Meet them with openness, acceptance, and equanimity. Whatever it is, it's okay to feel it. Be open to it.

3. **1-Minute Rest.** Take a 1-minute rest from the visualization, and practice mindful breathing.

4. **5 Minutes: Best-Case Scenario.** Visualize the very best-case scenario for this situation and simultaneously visualize yourself remaining equanimous throughout. Allow yourself to experience any physical sensations that occur as you imagine this scenario. You might feel a sense of spaciousness or lightness, or you might notice a change in your breathing. For some people, the physiology of pleasant anticipation can also manifest like anxiety: adrenaline may cause increased heart rate, perspiration, and a sense of lightness in the stomach. Let yourself move close to these sensations without trying to grasp at them. Greet them with openness, acceptance, and equanimity.

5. At the end of your practice, return your awareness to your breath and enjoy three full, conscious breaths. Gently wiggle your fingers and toes. Become aware of the space around you before you slowly open your eyes.

 PRACTICE TIPS

Practice each scenario in four separate sessions (ideally twice a day for two days) after your usual 20-minute meditation practice. After these four sessions, you'll be ready to approach the real-life situation with greater balance, calmness, and equanimity.

This practice allows you to prepare for challenging situations in a way that's radically different from your usual habits. You're learning how to dissolve patterns that keep you stuck in unhelpful behavioral cycles by staying present and open to both your own internal experience and the external situation, regardless of what occurs.

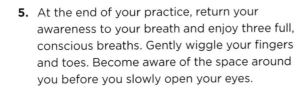

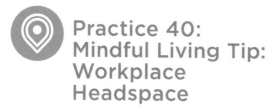

## Practice 40: Mindful Living Tip: Workplace Headspace

Here are four ways to bring more mindfulness to your workplace.

- **Meditate.** This may seem obvious, but it's important to say this explicitly. You can meditate at work! In fact, you can meditate anywhere and everywhere, and while it's true that some environments are more appealing than others, there's no real reason not to meditate at work. You might like to get to work early, or to sit at your desk wearing earphones so that no one will disturb you. You can also meditate in the bathroom, stairwell, or any other quiet area.

- **Be the change.** Research shows that mindfulness can be very beneficial in the workplace, but sadly, many organizations aren't yet offering meditation programs. Take the initiative, and coordinate a meditation group. You don't need much time—even 10 minutes will do—and you certainly don't need to be confident in guiding the group through a meditation yourself. Consider using one of the many great meditation apps or audios on the market, then press play and let an expert guide you and your group.

- **Practice mindfulness.** Formal meditation practice is essential—it's where the brain literally starts to rewire itself—but using mindfulness informally during daily life is a great way to experiment with and benefit from the skills you're cultivating. Apply any of the Mindful Living Tips from this book to your workplace. For example, you can use the mindful walking practice (see Practice 25) as you make your way from your desk to the water cooler, the elevator, or the bathroom.

- **Turn toward distractions.** Workplaces can be busy, chaotic places that are full of distractions, especially in open-plan offices, where phones, printers, conversations, and smartphone reminders are all competing for our attention. While our natural and habitual response might be to try to block things out, mindfulness meditation teaches us that, paradoxically, by allowing, paying attention, and opening our awareness to what's going on around us, we can press the reset button on our awareness, and refocus on whatever we choose to.

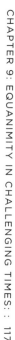

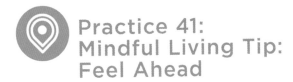

# Practice 41: Mindful Living Tip: Feel Ahead

Practicing mindfulness has been shown to enhance self-awareness and self-regulation, and this can translate into greater self-control and better performance when applied to the workplace. Here's a simple mindfulness practice that'll help you enhance these qualities and strengths.

## STEP 1

Take some time to look ahead at your schedule at the start of your workday. Before you begin, sit quietly and breathe for a few moments, tuning in to your body and bringing yourself into the present moment.

## STEP 2

As you take stock of your workday, allow yourself to "feel ahead." Notice any emotions and physical feelings that arise when you look at your schedule. Does your heart start to race when you contemplate that 2 p.m. meeting? Allow yourself to explore that further with curiosity and openness. Notice all of the physical sensations that come up; allow them to be there, then gently ask yourself what they're about. Are you experiencing excitement and eager anticipation when you think about that meeting, or are you filled with dread and anxiety about an announcement you need to make? Notice the storyline that develops in your mind about this situation. Simply observe whatever emerges in your body and mind.

Being aware of your feelings ahead of time allows you to be more mindful when you enter into the actual situation. You can use this feel ahead exercise to desensitize yourself to any unpleasant sensations that arise in relation to a certain situation. That way, when they occur again in the midst of the real event, you can choose to respond mindfully rather than react habitually. You can also use the feel ahead exercise to help you plan your day well. It might help you realize where you need to invest more time and energy, or it may give you insight into where you're procrastinating or overexpending energy.

## Practice 42: Mindful Living Tip: Monotasking

Research shows that multitasking wastes time; it slows you down, stresses you out, and ultimately makes you less productive. It turns out that our brains aren't really wired to multitask, and when we try to do so, we don't really multitask at all; we just switch rapidly between different tasks. We pay a high cognitive price for all this switching back and forth—including more stress and fatigue, and less efficiency and effectiveness.

Now that the detrimental effects of multitasking are clear, both mindfulness and monotasking (sometimes called unitasking) are gaining momentum, and they're close cousins. Mindfulness is the act of paying attention to the present moment, and monotasking is the act of doing one thing at a time. Each facilitates the other, and while both can be tricky to implement in the workplace, formal meditation practice will help. Here are a few extra tips for cultivating greater mindfulness through mono-tasking at work:

- **Keep things clear.** Clear the space around you so that you aren't distracted by different tasks. This might mean clearing your desk of the files and other items you're not using or closing other documents on your desktop.

- **Turn off and tune out.** Technology can be extremely distracting. Turn off your phone and email alerts during monotasking time.

- **Let it go.** If thoughts about other projects arise when you're focusing on something else, don't try to block them out, but don't indulge them, either. Let them be, but let them go. You might even like to thank your mind for the reminder, and tell yourself you'll get to it later.

- **Plan and prioritize.** Most people find that they're more productive at a particular time of day, so it's best to plan ahead and schedule intensive monotasking periods during these times. Prioritize your tasks weekly and day by day, so that you know you're investing time in the right things when you set yourself down to focus.

## Practice 43: Mindful Living Tip: Power-Down Hour

Another mini mind cleanse is the power-down hour, in which you disconnect from all things digital for 1 hour before bedtime. That means no mobile phones, iPads, or iPods; no computers, radio, or TV.

Like the mind cleanse on page 110, it's best to try the power-down hour for 2 weeks and then review your experience. If you find that the first thing you do each morning is reach for your mobile phone, then consider adding a power-down period to the start of your day. Checking social media or email upon waking means you miss out on the opportunity to begin your day with a mindful check-in.

The power-down hour has the added benefit of drawing our awareness to the rituals of how you end—and begin—your day. In doing this, many people discover that their well-being peaks when their habits are in sync with their natural circadian rhythms. Our ancient brains are attuned to this rhythm and to the movements of the Sun and Moon. We're hardwired to roam about during daylight hours and to sleep at night, and our bodies don't much like it when we violate that rhythm.

 It's humbling to remember that the majority of our grandparents' parents were still using gas lamps, as electric light only came into widespread use in the 1880s. Electricity and the technology that has followed it has had an enormous effect on our ability to violate our own circadian rhythms, which means we've taught ourselves to stay awake and stimulated for longer. This, in turn, disrupts the production of serotonin and other neurotransmitters that are critical to our physical and mental health. As you power-down in the evening (or morning), consider implementing other rituals that might help you live more mindfully.

# Practice 44: Mindful Living Tip: Social Stocktaking

In Practice 38, we explored the mind cleanse, a mindful living tip for becoming more conscious of what we feed our minds. Most people find that the mind cleanse heightens their awareness of the role that social media plays in their lives, and many are astounded by just how addictive it is.

In this practice, we'll delve further into social media addiction. We'll become more mindful of the factors that lead to it, and we'll explore a few ways to live mindfully amidst the technological mayhem of our contemporary lives.

## WHY ARE WE SO HOOKED ON SOCIAL MEDIA?

Most research has been done on why technology, and social media in particular, is so darn addictive. An entire book could be written on the topic—and it has!—so I'll summarize two of the key points here:

1. **We love novelty.** Our brains are hardwired to appreciate novelty, and new things capture our attention more easily than those we've already seen before. Evolutionary neuropsychologists have an explanation for this: They suggest that this tendency toward novelty was likely passed on because our ancestors who noticed new opportunities were more likely to thrive than those who didn't.

Today, our love of novelty is part of what makes scrolling around on the web so enticing. We can satisfy our craving for novelty without even leaving the couch.

2. **Watching, comparing, and contrasting— it's what we do.** We're also hardwired to compare and contrast ourselves to others in our social groups. This was both necessary and relatively easy for our ancestors, who compared themselves to the other individuals—usually about thirty people—in their immediate tribe. This would have helped them better understand their alliances with one another, feel secure, and get a sense of their roles within the group.

Today, we compare and contrast ourselves to an endless number of others—including people who live on the other side of the world, people we'll never meet in person, celebrities, and a whole host of other people who choose to share their lives on social media.

Combine our obsession with novelty with that drive to compare and contrast ourselves to others, and it's not hard to understand why we endlessly scroll through our social media accounts until we finally take our tired brains to bed.

## SO WHAT CAN WE DO?

Again, research has shown us that technology is addictive. That means we must set limits on what we allow our brains to consume. Left to their own devices, our brains will almost certainly consume, compare, and contrast themselves into exhausted, stressed-out messes. Mindful living means making the choice to take conscious, considered action.

- **Get clear.** Set some parameters around your use of social media. How much time do you want to spend on it, and when?

- **The cull.** Set aside some time to complete a stocktaking of your social media accounts. Assess the people and products you follow on social media, then make some cuts. If something or someone seldom adds anything positive or constructive to your life, then delete it (you can always add it again later, if you change your mind). If something makes you feel inferior, unworthy, uncentered, or uneasy, then delete for sure. Only feed your mind with nourishing food.

- **Digital detox.** Some people find it helpful to do a "cold turkey" digital detox, and to delete a particular app from their phones for a weekend or longer. For many, it's a liberating release! You can always reinstall the app later, if you like. In the meantime, enjoy the space for presence and mindfulness that opens up when that stubborn social media addiction is a just little further out of reach.

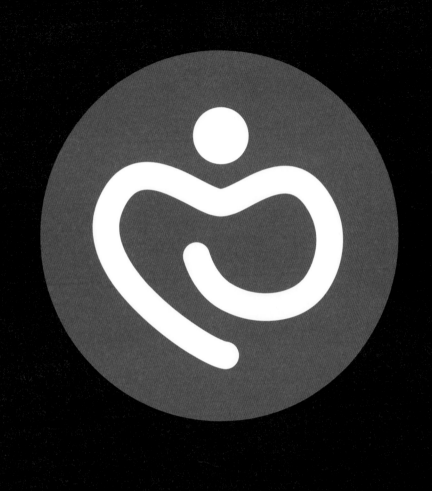

FROM THE PERSPECTIVE OF CONTEMPLATIVE TRADITIONS LIKE BUDDHISM, MEDITATION ISN'T ONLY ABOUT BECOMING LESS STRESSED, HEALTHIER, AND MORE PRODUCTIVE. ALTHOUGH THESE THINGS CERTAINLY DO HAPPEN—MEDITATION DOES ENABLE US TO BECOME MORE FOCUSED, LESS DISTRACTED, AND CALMER—MEDITATION IS, WAS, AND ALWAYS HAS BEEN ABOUT SOMETHING MORE. SOMETHING LESS EGOCENTRIC IN WHICH WE VIEW OURSELVES AS PART OF A WIDER HUMAN EXPERIENCE. SOMETHING THAT LOOKS, SOUNDS, AND FEELS LIKE LOVE.

## ❶ KEY CONCEPT: LOVING KINDNESS

Across the world's many philosophical, contemplative, and religious traditions, there seems to be agreement on at least a few things. Most of these traditions believe that **empathy**, **compassion**, and **love** are among the key core principles of wise living.

- **Empathy** concerns our capacity to understand and share another person's experience.
- **Compassion** is about our wish to relieve another's suffering.
- **Love** refers to a pervasive sense of connection and common humanity, based on the understanding that everyone (and everything) is interrelated.

Within Buddhist traditions, the three concepts of empathy, compassion, and love come together in a state known as *metta*, or **loving kindness**. Metta is a state in which a sense of deep interconnection, benevolence, and compassion pervades the mind as a way of being in which we hope for the happiness of ourselves and others. According to both Buddhist traditions and contemporary science, we're already hardwired for loving kindness, but if we wish to experience it to the full, we can and must cultivate it.

## THE SCIENCE OF COMPASSION

Until recently, little research had been done on the human potential for cultivating compassion. Forty years of meditation research has largely focused on the way in which meditation practices induce relaxation and enhance mindfulness, but what about the effects of meditation techniques that were intended for cultivating compassion? Thankfully, over the past decade, interest in this field has flourished, and traditional meditation practices for cultivating loving kindness and compassion have been researched in laboratory settings. Studies show that these practices have a unique effect on the parts of the brain that are associated with empathy, emotional perception, and sensitivity.

Interestingly (and encouragingly), the research also suggests that you don't need years of practice to enhance your capacity for loving kindness and compassion. In fact, practicing just 10 minutes of loving kindness meditation can increase feelings of social connection and positivity toward others. In a paper published in 2013 in the journal *Psychological Science*, researchers assigned participants to a 30-minute guided audio practice, which they listened to each day for 2 weeks. Half of the participants listened to a guided loving kindness meditation, while the other half listened to a reappraisal training technique that taught them to think about stressful experiences in new, less upsetting ways, including considering events from another person's point of view. Before and immediately after the 2-week training, all participants underwent functional MRI brain scans while they looked at a series of images, some of which depicted people in pain (such as a burn victim or a distressed child). The study demonstrated that meditators exhibited more changes in the regions of the brain that are associated with empathy, emotional regulation, and positive emotions.

---

True to its name, **loving kindness** is a form of love that's characterized by kindness. It's valued and practiced across a wide range of religious traditions.

---

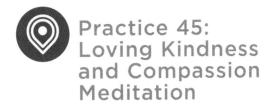

# Practice 45: Loving Kindness and Compassion Meditation

This meditation activates and cultivates your inherent qualities of tenderness, care, concern, warmth, openheartedness, and empathy. It's a great daily practice—and it's also a beautiful balm you can apply when you're feeling lonely, separate from others, or hardened to yourself or the world.

## TECHNIQUE

1. Sit in any position that's comfortable for you and close your eyes. (It's important to be physically comfortable here, so take a moment to relax any parts of your body that are especially tense.)

2. Begin by gently moving your attention to the process of breathing. Enjoy three full, deep, conscious breaths. Then allow your breath to settle into a natural rhythm. Allow the breath to breathe itself.

3. Draw your inner gaze to the area of your heart.

4. **A Loved One.** Now bring to mind someone you love very much. As you inhale, feel the area around your heart expand, and allow this love to permeate your body. You might wish to visualize this love as a golden stream of light emanating to and from your heart. As you exhale, gradually expand and extend these positive, loving, compassionate, benevolent thoughts toward your loved one. Silently recite the following phrases, or say in your own words: *"May you have happiness, joy, and peace. May you be free from suffering. May you experience love."*

5. **Yourself.** With your awareness centered in your heart, bring loving kindness toward yourself. As you inhale, feel the area around your heart expand, and allow this love to permeate your body. As you exhale, gradually expand and extend these positive, loving, compassionate, benevolent thoughts toward yourself. Silently recite the following phrases, or say in your own words: *"May I have happiness, joy, and peace. May I be free from suffering. May I experience love."*

6. **A Stranger.** Now, visualize someone toward whom you have neutral feelings—someone you may see in your daily life but who you don't know, such as a bus driver or a classmate. Bring your awareness to your heart and extend the light of love, kindness, and compassion from your heart to her or him, with the message: *"May you have happiness, joy, and peace. May you be free from suffering. May you experience love."*

7. **An "Enemy."** This time, visualize a person with whom you've had some kind of conflict. Extend the light of love, kindness, and compassion from your heart to him or her, with the message: *"May you have happiness, joy, and peace. May you be free from suffering. May you experience love."*

8. **All Beings.** Let your awareness and love rove further. As you inhale, feel the area around your heart expand, and allow this love to permeate your body. As you exhale, gradually expand and extend these positive, loving, compassionate, benevolent thoughts toward all beings. Bring to mind acquaintances, colleagues, neighbors, and other people in your community. Include those with whom you may have had conflict. Now expand and extend your kindness and your loving wishes to the entire world and all beings within it, including animals. Inhale and feel your heart expand. Exhale, and let these positive qualities radiate from you and within you. Continue for as long as you wish.

9. **Rest.** Rest in the joy of opening your heart in this way.

10. At the end of your practice, take a few moments to expand your awareness from the breath into the room around you. When you feel ready, open your eyes.

 **PRACTICE TIPS**

- Practice daily for 10 to 20 minutes.

- Don't worry if you struggle to extend your loving kindness to challenging people (or to yourself). Try to remain calm, stable, and spacious, and work your way in gently. It's okay to back off if it's too much. In that case, try this helpful practice: Reflect on the other person (or yourself), and visualize her or him as an infant or young child.

- Once you're familiar with this meditation, you can practice a shorter, 5-minute version of it at the end of any meditation practice.

## Practice 46: The View

There are many ways to experience a sense of our interconnectedness and shared humanity. In fact, the idea and practice of extending our awareness to comprehend the interrelatedness of life is one that's shared by scientists as well as religious and contemplative practitioners. Albert Einstein, one of the world's great scientists, professed a profound sense of interconnectedness with the world around him. In 1972, the *New York Times* published a letter he had written to his friend in 1950.

**"A human being is a part of the whole called by us 'the universe,' a part limited in time and space. He experiences himself, his thoughts and feelings, as something separate from the rest—a kind of optical illusion of consciousness. This delusion is a kind of prison for us, restricting us to our personal desires and affection for a few persons nearest to us. Our task must be to free ourselves from this prison by widening the circle of understanding and compassion to embrace all living creatures and the whole of nature in its beauty."**

During the same era in which Einstein's letter was published, we got the first glimpses of how our planet looks from outer space—that is, from the perspective of the cosmos. It was awe-inspiring, particularly for the astronauts who captured these images. Many of them came to experience something known as the overview effect—a profound shift in perspective and awareness characterized by a sense of awe, a deep sense of the interconnectedness of life, and a strong sense of responsibility to care for all living things.

Happily, we don't need to launch ourselves into outer space to experience such expansive, heart-opening sentiments. Through meditation and contemplation, we are all able to free ourselves from the "optical illusion of consciousness," to use Einstein's phrase, and to extend our vision and compassion to the world as a whole.

### TECHNIQUE

1. Sit in any position that's comfortable for you and close your eyes.

2. Enjoy three full, slow, deep breaths. Fill the abdomen as you inhale and allow your entire body to soften as you exhale. Then allow your breath to settle into a natural rhythm.

3. Ground yourself here in the present moment by connecting with each of your five senses: revisit the five senses practice on page 28, if you like.

4. Now, in your mind's eye, visualize yourself sitting in the room you're in. Take note of everything you can see. Notice the furniture in the room; notice the clothing you're wearing; and travel around your body to see yourself from different angles.

5. Once you have a clear image in your mind's eye of yourself in the room, shift your perspective and imagine that you're looking at yourself from outside or above the building you're in.

6. Continue to hover and expand your perspective. View yourself in your mind's eye from an ever-increasing distance. See yourself within your building, within your neighborhood.

7. Keep on extending and expanding your view. See yourself within your community, your city, state, country, continent, and, eventually, this planet.

8. Let your awareness hover about this planet, and contemplate the pulsing rhythm of life below and the vastness and interconnectedness of all life. Take a moment to extend your deepest aspirations for the world, for all of humanity. You might say to yourself, "May peace prevail," "The world is filled with love," "May all beings be happy," "We are all connected through love," or any other phrase that resonates with you.

9. Travel even farther away from Earth, seeing it as one of many within this galaxy. Contemplate the enormity, vastness, and expansiveness of life.

10. When you're ready to complete this practice, slowly transition back into your body. Gradually return from the cosmos to the Earth, then your continent, country, state, city, neighborhood, building, and room. Take a few moments to expand your awareness back into your five senses: sound, taste, smell, touch, and sight. Feel the presence of your physical body in this room. When you feel ready, open your eyes.

 PRACTICE TIP

Practice daily for 10 to 20 minutes.

## Practice 47: Tonglen

*Tonglen*—which means "giving and taking" or "sending and receiving"—is a meditation practice from the Tibetan tradition. Like the loving kindness and compassion meditation (see Practice 45), it too encourages us to connect with others, but *tonglen* invites us directly into the tender heart of suffering and compassion. We develop our ability to perceive and be present with our own suffering and that of others. In this way, that which we usually resent, resist, or ignore—the presence of suffering—becomes a tool to help us open our minds and hearts.

The practice involves breathing in the pain of others, along with the wish to relieve their suffering, followed by an exhalation of happiness, joy, and love that's intended to bring them relief. It can also provide us with the valuable opportunity to tune in to and overcome any internal obstacles that might be preventing us from experiencing and expressing empathy and compassion. In recognizing that others suffer just as we do, we ignite our kindness and openness.

Tonglen is a rich practice—but it's a tender one, too. It can feel overwhelming for some people, so it's best to practice it only when you feel comfortable enough to do so. But during the times at which you feel powerless in the face of the world's suffering, remember that there is something you can do to help: You can practice tonglen. As the Dalai Lama has said, "Whether this [tonglen] meditation really helps others or not, it gives me peace of mind. Then I can be more effective, and the benefit is immense." It's true: the practice is equally beneficial when you're suffering or feeling isolated yourself, and it's also a brilliant antidote to self-pity. Self-pity is not the same thing as self-compassion. According to self-compassion researcher Dr. Kristin Neff, self-pity tends to be more egocentric and ignores the interconnected nature of our suffering (and our happiness). It can also overemphasize and exaggerate our personal struggles. In contrast, self-compassion arises from the intent to be loving. It invites us to into a mind space in which the broader context of our shared human suffering is held in perspective. The practice of tonglen is one way to reverse the flow of ego, and to transform such thinking into true compassion and equanimity.

## TECHNIQUE

1. Always begin by meditating first, using your favorite practice.

2. **A Loved One.** Begin tonglen by bringing to mind someone whom you know and want to help, such as a child who's struggling at school, a friend who's experiencing a relationship problem, or a family member who's suffering from depression.

3. As you inhale, take in the heaviness of his suffering, giving him space for relief and healing. It's not necessary to have a specific word to describe the suffering: it can simply be a feeling, perhaps of darkness, heat, or heaviness.

4. Breathe out love, peace, or any other positive idea that you believe would bring him comfort. Let your kindness and compassionate love fill him. You might like to visualize this out-breath as white in color, or cool in temperature.

5. **Yourself.** Now contemplate your own physical or emotional suffering, and consider that you're not alone—other people feel like this, too. Allow your inhalation to absorb this suffering from yourself and others. As you exhale, extend the heartfelt wish that both you and others might be free from this suffering.

6. **A Stranger.** Now visualize someone toward whom you have neutral feelings, perhaps a bus driver or a classmate. Even though you don't know the details of this person's life, imagine how she has suffered or struggled at times—just like you have.

7. As you inhale, take in the heaviness of her suffering, giving her space for relief and healing. Breathe out love, peace, or any other positive idea that you believe would bring her comfort.

8. **An "Enemy."** This time, visualize someone with whom you've had some kind of conflict. Even though you might have some negative feelings toward this person, imagine how he has suffered or struggled at times—just like you have. Consider that he wants to be happy—just like you do.

9. As you inhale, take in the heaviness of his suffering, giving him space for relief and healing. Breathe out love, peace, or any other positive idea that you believe would bring him comfort.

10. **All Beings.** Now contemplate the suffering of the world and of all beings: those who suffer from poverty, injustices, and the afflictions of their own minds. Contemplate your aspiration for the world and humanity. As you breathe in, take in the heaviness of this suffering. As you exhale, extend your genuine wish that all beings might feel at peace.

11. **Rest.** Continue to breathe with full awareness, and let your loving intentions keep on radiating outward. Allow any residual heaviness and suffering to be transformed by this love.

12. Rest for a few moments in this vast openness of love and peace. (You don't need to call anyone or anything specific to mind here: simply continue to breathe.)

13. At the end of your practice, take a few moments to expand your awareness from the breath into the room around you. Become aware of your body, and gently wiggle your fingers and toes. When you feel ready, slowly open your eyes.

##  PRACTICE TIPS

- Practice daily for 10 to 20 minutes.

- Don't worry that breathing in suffering means that suffering will become a part of you. There is no evidence that this practice will decrease or deplete your own well-being.

- If you feel blocked or stuck in this practice at any point—perhaps through resistance, anger, shame, or discomfort—change the focus of the meditation. Instead of contemplating another's pain or suffering, tune in to what you're feeling in the present moment. Complete the practice for yourself and for all others who are feeling or have felt just like you do in this moment.

### SPOTLIGHT ON SCIENCE

There are few stand-alone scientific studies of *tonglen*: to date, most have explored Loving Kindness meditation or a combination or the two. But in 2014, the first empirical study of *tonglen* investigated changes in compassion and found an increase in self-compassion as well as a sense of common shared humanity after only 6 days of practice.

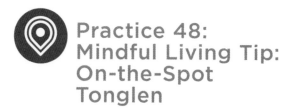

# Practice 48:
# Mindful Living Tip:
# On-the-Spot
# Tonglen

Once you are familiar with the formal practice of *tonglen* (see Practice 47), you can begin to take this heart-opening practice with you into everyday life.

Informal *tonglen* can be practiced on the spot—in any spot. You can do it while you're sitting beside someone who's ill, dying, or who has just died, or while you see someone in pain while you're walking down the street. Notice the world around you. You might become aware of the stress, unhappiness, fatigue, or anger on the faces of people next to you on the train, bus, or elevator. Allow yourself to open up, to empathize with them, and to share a little of their pain and suffering.

## Practice 49: Mindful Living Tip: Compassion in Action

As you activate the empathy networks within your brain through the practices in chapter 10, you might find that you wish to help people in other ways, too. This "kindness urge" arises through empathy and compassion—and it's important to act on it. Go ahead and move your compassion into action, and allow yourself to express and explore your potential for kindness.

Start by considering acts of kindness. Make a list of things you could do for another person (either someone you know or a stranger) that would bring joy to him or her. This doesn't have to be complicated. It might be as simple as sending a card to a friend, cooking a meal for someone you know, offering to help with a task, or pushing past the hesitation to give your small change to someone who is homeless.

Make a list of the things you could do, and get ready to do them (for example, gather your small change and put it into your right pocket so you're all set to donate it to the homeless man you see each evening; or buy some cards so that you have them on hand when you need them). Then make a note in your diary to perform an act of kindness each week or month until this new pattern becomes habit. You'll soon find yourself expressing more and more of the love, kindness, and compassion that already lies within you.

### SPOTLIGHT ON SCIENCE

Research supports the notion that different meditation styles do different things and are characterized by different patterns of neural activation. However, this research is still in its infancy and it's too early to definitively say which approach to meditation is best for any given person at a particular point in time. The best advice is to explore different techniques and find out what works better for you.

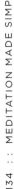

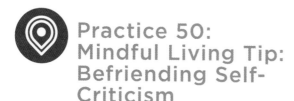

# Practice 50: Mindful Living Tip: Befriending Self-Criticism

Self-compassion is good for you. According to a number of studies, it correlates with greater psychological health, lower levels of anxiety and depression, and less stress, rumination, and perfectionism.

Mindfulness strengthens our capacity for self-compassion as well as our metacognition or our ability to think about our own thinking. Significantly, research suggests that self-compassionate people don't try to suppress negative thoughts. Instead, they acknowledge and accept their negative thoughts and emotions and appear to defuse these experiences from causing further difficulty by accepting them.

The loving kindness and tonglen meditations in this chapter have been shown to increase self-compassion, and this mindful living tip offers extra tools for befriending yourself by bringing compassion to your negative thoughts.

## STEP 1: WATCH THE CRITIC

Begin by paying attention to your internal critic—that voice in your head that seems to judge so much of what you do. What do you tend to criticize yourself for? Write down the issues that come up. Now that you've observed your self-critical thoughts, allow yourself to see them for what they are—just thoughts. These thoughts might also give you clues about their origins; perhaps the voice in which they're articulated is very like that of a person from your past. Do these thoughts remind you of anyone or of a particular situation?

## STEP 2: SOFTEN THE STORY

Now begin to soften to and around the self-critical voice. To start, it might be helpful to imagine how you would respond to a friend who was expressing these thoughts and beliefs. How would you react? Would you be harsh and judgmental about the fact that she's having critical thoughts—or would you tell her that it's okay to have such thoughts, but that it doesn't mean they're true?

It's important both to accept the self-critical thoughts and to soften and balance them with insight and wisdom. For instance, you might respond to yourself by saying, "Thank you, mind! I know you're worried about me, but your message is actually causing extra and unnecessary suffering. I know I can handle this situation, no matter what the outcome is."

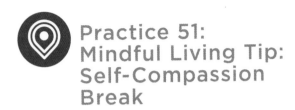

## Practice 51: Mindful Living Tip: Self-Compassion Break

Compassion for oneself and compassion for others are two sides of the same coin. Both require mindfulness, which strengthens your ability to remain present to any experience with acceptance and equanimity. Both also require empathy—your ability and willingness to turn toward and understand your own experience or that of another person. Together, this combination of mindful presence and empathy lays the groundwork for compassion: the wish and intention to relieve your own suffering and the suffering of others.

Many people report that they find practicing self-compassion much more challenging than practicing compassion toward others, but this short exercise can help. It encourages you to extend your capacity for compassion toward yourself—even in the heat of the moment, when you feel angry, frustrated, disappointed, or judgmental—and it just takes 3 minutes of mindful contemplation.

### MINUTE 1: ACKNOWLEDGE THIS MOMENT OF SUFFERING

Allow yourself to feel into what's happening for you right now, whether it's physical pain, stress, shame, or anger. Be present to the fact that this is a moment in which you are experiencing some kind of pain.

### MINUTE 2: ACKNOWLEDGE AND ACCEPT PERSONAL AND COLLECTIVE SUFFERING

Everyone feels pain. You are not alone in this experience—not even in this particular moment. There are more than 7 billion people on this planet, and every single one of them experiences suffering at some point. In fact, someone else is suffering right now, just as you are. Contemplate this and cultivate a sense of shared humanity and shared suffering.

### MINUTE 3: CULTIVATE KINDNESS

Think about what you really need in this moment. What is the wisest, kindest thing you need to hear or do right now? You might want to extend a heartfelt wish to yourself, such as "May I be kind, forgiving, patient, and compassionate to myself." You could also consider how you'd respond to a friend in a similar situation. How would you demonstrate kindness and compassion to him? What would you say to her? What would you do for them?

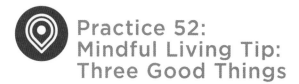 ## Practice 52: Mindful Living Tip: Three Good Things

It's not always easy to focus on the goodness and greatness in life. For most of us, it's a skill we have to cultivate actively and curate mindfully. This peculiar human challenge is explained by something neuroscientists call the "negativity bias." Because of this brain bias, we're hardwired to notice and remember negative information more than positive information.

Our negativity bias may be inconvenient, but it's no mistake. From an evolutionary perspective, it makes good sense. Ancestors of ours who were tuned in to any and all potential sources of threat were more likely to survive than those who were blissfully ignorant. It is one of our species' great evolutionary assets.

However, the negativity bias is also part of what makes it so hard to notice all the good stuff that's going on around us. It's part of what makes it difficult to be in the present moment in a loving and open way, particularly when we face an onslaught of negative news and information in the media (not to mention the stressors in our own lives). That's why it's important to remember that a "positivity bias" is something we can, and must, cultivate. Here's how.

## PRACTICE "THREE GOOD THINGS"

Set aside time at the end of each day to recall three good things about your day. This might surprise you—even if you feel like you had a terrible day, you're sure to discover three things at the very least! You might find yourself recalling with gratitude the barista's warm smile as he handed you your morning coffee, a kind word from a colleague, or the beautiful sunset you saw as you were driving home.

This three good things practice can be performed in silent contemplation, written in a journal, or spoken aloud to another person. (It can be especially wonderful to share your three good things with your partner or another loved one.)

This practice takes only a few seconds, but research has shown that it's one of the easiest and most effective tools for boosting happiness and fostering a sense of gratitude.

# Summary

Congratulations! You've explored fifty-two practices for optimizing your brain function, cultivating your mind, and opening your heart, and you've expanded your awareness—which is to say, your consciousness—on this journey.

Of course, you haven't learned to do anything you didn't already know how to do. You already had an inherent ability to be present, open, curious, expansive, kind, connected, compassionate, and loving. Now you know how to enhance these qualities and to step past the cacophony in your busy, everyday mind to experience the more expansive aspects of yourself.

It's time to curate your own meditation and mindfulness practice. You've learned both formal meditation practices and informal strategies for mindful living, and most people find that a combination of the two yields the most benefits. Here are some key tips for using the techniques covered in this book:

- **Begin mindfully.** Begin your day, your workday, and each activity by taking a moment to center and ground yourself in the present moment.

- **Befriend breath.** Your breath is both a measure of the state of your nervous system and your tool for calming and de-stressing it. Become familiar with tuning in to your breath, and practice releasing tension through conscious breathing.

- **Apply as needed.** Mindfulness tools can be used everywhere, even in emergencies. Use the 3-minute mind shower on page 77 whenever you're feeling overwhelmed. Punctuate your day with this handy method for checking in, tuning in, and calming down.

- **Awareness, acceptance, compassion, patience, persistence—and a healthy dose of humor.** The mindful way of living unfolds as a process. It doesn't happen overnight (although moments of complete presence can, and do, happen within any moment). The key concepts or attitudes of mindfulness detailed in each chapter of this book are your allies. They can help you transform old, habitual patterns of reaction and awaken to alternative ways of being.

- **Practice.** Both formal and informal practices are essential for maximizing the benefits of meditation and mindfulness. Try your best to commit to a daily ritual that incorporates your favorite formal meditation practice(s).

## YOUR CUSTOM-MADE PRACTICE

It's as true for meditation as it is for clothes: "one size fits all" never fits everyone. That's why I encourage an approach I call "bespoke" or "custom-made" meditation.

Interestingly, this approach is also found in India, where there are many different pathways to meditation. The great Indian yoga teacher T. K. V. Desikachar addressed the need for bespoke practices:

> "Anybody who wants to can practice yoga. Anybody can breathe; therefore anybody can practice yoga. But no one can practice every kind of yoga. It has to be the right yoga for the person. The student and teacher meet and decide on a program that is acceptable and suitable to that person."

Ditto for meditation, which Indian tradition views as a branch of the "tree" of yoga.

A great deal of Western scientific research has explored meditation in recent decades, and a thriving little meditation industry has also been gaining momentum. The science behind it is sound: meditation is good for us and, as I see it, public interest in meditation is a great thing. It's great for individuals, and it's great for communities, too. But it's also a plus for those who have a vested interest in acquainting you with meditation. Whether that interest is financial, political, philosophical, or otherwise, the truth is that members of the industry do stand to gain by convincing you that their particular meditation technique is "the best"—and that it's the best for you, specifically.

As both a clinical psychologist and a meditation teacher, I use meditation as a big part of my work. This means that I'm one of the people who stands to gain from advocating a particular practice—yet my scientific training (as well as my training in contemplative and yogic traditions) has taught me that no one particular meditation technique can claim to be the best for everyone.

Some approaches have received more attention than others from the scientific community, and some have received more celebrity endorsements. Current neuroscience also indicates that we'll probably learn more about the advantages of different techniques in the future—and for whom, and when, they're most effective, but the fact is, we just don't know enough to make these claims yet.

I've worked with clients who, like the proverbial square peg in a round hole, literally forced themselves to practice meditation techniques that really didn't fit their situations or constitutions—and that's counterproductive. After all, no one assumes that one type of exercise is the best approach for everyone: just as we all have unique physical constitutions, we also have different neurological profiles. Our personalities are different, as are our environments and our beliefs. We pass through different life stages and phases, and honestly, we all come to meditation with different needs, goals, and intentions.

I've seen many clients who have been referred by their GPs for help with stress and anxiety. In conjunction with cognitive behavioral therapy (CBT), meditation has been shown to reduce relapse rates in depression, and an increasing number of my clients hope to safely manage their risk of relapse while reducing their reliance on antidepressants. Others aim to improve their ability to focus, pay attention, and be present in their jobs and with their loved ones. Still others want to be less angry (meaning less reactive). Some are responding to an inner calling that's drawing them to deepen their personal spiritual practices. One thing is for sure: *one size will not fit all of them.*

Some people are drawn to "purist" paths and orthodox traditions within meditation. They find wisdom in complete commitment and devotion to one philosophy, one approach, one way of being in this world. People certainly can (and do) take an orthodox perspective on different meditation techniques, but, as in all traditions, the orthodox approach tends to really suit only a minority of individuals. Don't get me wrong, we need orthodox traditions: they keep the techniques pure, and we return to such teachers for knowledge because they've been immersed in their methods so intently and intensively. It's a beautiful path, but it's not for everyone.

Many folks aren't orthodox. They're integrators (or perhaps instigators), and they're synthesizers, too. They might even be able to comprehend the ways in which all orthodox traditions interrelate, and they may find profound meaning in this oneness. They synthesize, and, as in the biological world, they hybridize until they find what works for them, in their world, right now (knowing that that will probably change in the future). They find themselves asking questions, such as, "Can we be both audaciously original and profoundly respectful of the traditions from which we have borrowed? Can we imbibe contemplative wisdom and apply it meaningfully, creatively, and usefully in our modern lives?"

There are many paths to meditation because we need them. By now, you've learned dozens of different methods, and a little bit about the current scientific research that supports their value. Now, I encourage you to follow your own path. This book is an invitation to play and experiment with these practices, and I hope you'll accept that invitation. I hope you'll notice what enlivens you and then explore it further. Above all, I hope this book has planted a seed that will draw you into a new intimacy with yourself and a new way of connecting with others and the world around you.

# Q&A

This is your guide to common questions and concerns about meditation.

## MY MIND KEEPS WANDERING.

Not only is this completely normal, but it's also what's supposed to happen. Remember: It's the nature of the heart to beat, and it's the nature of the mind to think. When you realize your mind has wandered off, all you need to do is come back to the object of your meditation and start again. Don't worry: you are practicing correctly. This repetitive activity is part of what helps activate the relaxation response in your body.

You don't need to stop your thoughts or to analyze them. Just be neutral toward them. Keep on returning your awareness to the object of your meditation without force or strain. Strange or random thoughts and images are completely normal, too. As you move out of your "doing" mode, your mind will journey into other levels of awareness. Don't engage with the content of these thoughts; Just let them be but let them go, and float your awareness back to the object of your meditation.

## HOW DO I KNOW IF IT'S WORKING?

Never judge an individual meditation session. Always measure your meditation by the benefits it brings to your day-to-day life.

## I CAN'T SIT STILL!

If you're feeling restless, check to see if there's something that could be revving up your mind and body. Have you just consumed caffeine or sugar? If so, try avoiding these stimulants for a couple of hours before your next meditation practice.

It's also important to know that there will be times when your mind is simply agitated and restless, particularly if you're experiencing stress. Relaxation can seem impossible when you're stressed, overstimulated, or anxious, and sometimes you might feel restless for your entire meditation practice. That's okay. Your meditation practice will still be beneficial; you'll still have released stress, even if you don't feel as if you have. The more you stop trying to resist the restlessness, the more your mind will move beyond it.

## I GET SLEEPY.

Don't be concerned if you fall asleep during meditation. This will happen to almost all meditators at some point. In part, that's because our contemporary fast-paced lifestyles lead to fatigue. If you're not getting enough rest (and most people aren't), then your tired brain and body will view meditation as an opportunity for some much-needed repair time. That's okay. Be gentle with yourself. Remember that whatever is happening during meditation is not to be judged. There will be times when taking a nap is the most profoundly nourishing thing you can do for yourself. As you continue to release fatigue and counteract stress through daily meditation, you'll become less and less fatigued over time.

If fatigue continues, then it might be time to consider going to bed earlier or making other lifestyle changes. Take a look at your diet, blood sugar levels, and caffeine intake. Meditation has the extraordinary ability to bring mindfulness to all areas of our lives.

Alternatively, practicing at a different time of the day might help. Late in the evening probably isn't going to be a good idea, so try practicing in the morning or afternoon. Open a window to give yourself some fresh air. Good posture can help, too. Try to sit upright without using any back support. Keep your neck straight and your chin slightly lifted to avoid that droopy, dozing-head position.

Sometimes your meditation practice will be very deep, and it can be hard to come out of it. Try some gentle stretches at the end of your practice before you open your eyes. If you still feel groggy after your practice, splash some water on your face, or walk around outside and get some fresh air. If you have the luxury of time at your disposal, enjoy a power nap after your meditation practice.

## EVERY PRACTICE IS DIFFERENT.

Every meditation session will be different. It may be deep or shallow, calm or restless, gratifying or ungratifying. No one particular experience is better than another, and there's no such thing as a bad meditation. Whether it's shallow, restless, thought filled, or ungratifying, meditation plays an important role in releasing stress and allows us to practice remaining equanimous to all experiences.

Let go of expectations or preferences, and be open to your current experience as it is. When you notice yourself judging your meditation practice or trying to control what you are experiencing during meditation, let go of the judgment and simply come back to your object of meditation.

## I'M UNCOMFORTABLE.

If you become physically uncomfortable during meditation, simply reposition yourself until you're comfy again. Gently stretch if you need to, then settle into your meditation once again.

## I HAVE STRANGE BODY SENSATIONS.

You can experience a broad range of physical sensations during meditation.

### NUMBNESS/HEAVINESS

It's not uncommon to lose a sense of your hands or feet (or even your whole body) during meditation. Sometimes, the body can feel heavy or even numb. Don't worry: this is completely normal, and is simply an indication that you're becoming deeply relaxed. Simply allow this experience to happen. Your normal sensations will return when you come out of deep relaxation.

### NAUSEA/DIZZINESS

If the sensation is not overwhelming, float your awareness back to the object of meditation. If it does become overwhelming, you might wish to lie down on your back and just breathe until you feel able to sit upright again.

### TWITCHING/TINGLING/PRESSURE

The body expresses involuntary movements all the time, and during meditation, we can become more aware of these experiences. Some of these movements and sensations might have been happening all along; you simply may not have noticed them until now. It's similar to the way in which people often report that they have more thoughts since they started meditating, when in fact they're just more aware of their minds. When you find your attention has been drawn to some physical sensation, simply take note of it and then gently return your awareness to the object of meditation. The sensation will pass, and yes, sensations are a normal experience in meditation.

It's also not uncommon for old memories to arise when we enter into a deeply relaxed state. These memories can be accompanied by physical sensations. Don't be alarmed. Some people do experience quite unfamiliar twitching, shaking, pulsing, or aching sensations during meditation. This is because emotions are psychophysiological events—they dwell in both the mind and the body. Emotional memories are often accompanied by strong physical sensations. Try not to avoid, deny, block, or push away these experiences. Allow them to be there while you continue to gently guide your attention back to the breath. If you find yourself working with intensely difficult memories, sensations, and emotions, then it's important to seek support. Find a registered psychologist who is also trained in mindfulness approaches.

## HOW DO I MAKE MEDITATION A HABIT?

Initiating a new habit can be challenging, but the good news is that the very practice of meditation helps you rewire new neural pathways, which will assist you in developing new habits and breaking old ones. Here are some more tips for making meditation a daily habit:

- **Plan ahead.** Make meditation a key priority in your life. Think of your meditation time as a nonnegotiable meeting with yourself. Try not to skip it.

- **Be reasonable.** Set yourself up for success by setting aside a reasonable time frame for meditation. Start with a small, realistic, achievable time frame, such as 5 to 15 minutes.

- **Set reminders.** Set a reminder on your smartphone for 5 minutes before your meditation session so you can start to get organized and wind down for your practice.

- **Seek support.** Ask a friend to help you stay on track. Just like an exercise or gym buddy, a mediation buddy can help you stay accountable and committed to your meditation practice.

- **Know your why.** People meditate for different reasons, but most do so because they want to be the very best versions of themselves. Get clear about why you're making meditation a daily habit. What's your reason? Why is meditation important to you? Perhaps you want to be more present with your partner, less reactive to your children, or more empathic with others. Maybe you want to deepen your connection to your sense of purpose, or simply lower your blood pressure. Whatever it is, articulate it to yourself.

- **Be kind.** If it's been a few days (or even weeks) since your last meditation session, don't compound the situation with negative self-talk, guilt, and blame. Let it go and reset. You might like to explore what led to your lapse, and to plan ways to avoid similar scenarios in the future.

## WHY DO I HAVE THE THOUGHTS THAT I DO DURING MEDITATION?

The brain is always busy, even when we're at rest. Neurons are always connecting with each other, and we're thinking most of the time. There are two main contexts that can trigger specific types of thoughts: one is external, and the other is internal.

External triggers for thoughts are stimuli that happen in our environment. The smell of the bread your neighbor is baking might remind you of your grandmother, or the sound of screeching car breaks might trigger a memory of a long-ago car accident. Our brains (and senses) are hardwired to be attuned to our environment, and this is why meditating in a quiet environment is more conducive to quieting the mind.

The origin of thoughts triggered by internal experiences can be harder to detect. For one thing, thoughts can be triggered by physical sensations. For example, a sharp sensation in a tooth might be followed by thoughts about how long it's been since you've been to the dentist. Other body sensations might be subtler, and some can trigger very deeply held and even traumatic memories. Thoughts and memories themselves are internal experiences that can trigger further thoughts.

Three additional factors may influence why certain thoughts—that is to say, certain neural networks—are more likely to be triggered than others: *recency, frequency,* and *intensity.* The more *recently* or *frequently* a particular thought or idea has occurred, the more it's likely to arise again, particularly as we begin to relax and meditate. For example, if you watch the news before beginning your meditation practice, then it's likely that images or ideas about what you witnessed will crop up as your brain processes the information. Similarly, if you're working on a big project and have been thinking about a particular topic frequently over recent weeks, then those neural networks will be all fired up, and it's likely you'll find yourself thinking about it again. *Intensity* also plays a role, which means that thoughts or memories with a strong emotional tone are more easily generated.

In meditation, we cease to respond to the activation of neural networks with further activation. In other words, we stop responding to a particular thought or pattern of thoughts by continuing to think about it. Gradually, the strength of these thoughts decreases. When thoughts are no longer generated in response to preceding thoughts, older thought patterns (or weaker neural connections) may be activated. This is commonly experienced in meditation when older memories arise.

Memories with a stronger emotional tone or intensity appear to have stronger neural connections and are more resistant to the passage of time. From an evolutionary perspective, it's understandable that we'd easily retain and recall memories that remind us of things that once threatened our well-being, since we could learn from those events, draw on our experiences with them, and find ways to outwit them in the future.

It's important to remember that meditation is not concerned with analyzing the *content* of our thoughts. That's psychotherapy's job. The two practices do work in tandem and share many features, but one key difference is that psychotherapy focuses more on the content of the thoughts themselves, while meditation goes beyond them.

## Acknowledgments

To Remy, who lived in my belly as I wrote this book.

## About the Author

Dr. Paula Watkins is a clinical psychologist, meditation teacher, and mother. As one of Australia's leading meditation experts, she brings together her knowledge of psychology, meditation, neuroscience, and yoga to help people transform their brains, bodies, minds, hearts, and lives by pairing authentic teachings with cutting-edge science. She is the founder of Calm, Conscious & Connected, the first online meditation course pairing traditional practices with scientific research. She lives by the beach in Australia but still calls New Zealand home.

# References

## CHAPTER 1

Fareedabanu, A., B. Shetty, and P. Darshit. "A Comparative Study of Effect of Nadi-Shodhan Pranayama and Suryanamaskar on Pulmonary Functions." *Indian Journal of Ancient Medicine and Yoga* 5, no. 3 (2012): 121.

Keuning, J. "On the Nasal Cycle." *International Rhinology* 6 (1968): 99–136.

Klein, R., D. Pilon, S. Prosser, and D. Shannahoff-Khalsa. "Nasal Airflow Asymmetries and Human Performance." *Biological Psychology* 23 (1986): 127–137.

Marshall, R. S., A. Basilakos, T. Williams, and K. Love-Myers. "Exploring the Benefits of Unilateral Nostril Breathing Practice Post-Stroke: Attention, Language, Spatial Abilities, Depression, and Anxiety." *The Journal of Alternative and Complementary Medicine* 20, no. 3 (2014): 185–194.

Martin, G. N. *The Neuropsychology of Smell and Taste.* New York: Routledge, 2013.

Schiff, B. B., and S. A. Rump. "Asymmetrical Hemispheric Activation and Emotion—the Effects of Unilateral Forced Nostril Breathing." *Brain and Cognition* 29, no. 3 (1995): 217–231.

Shannahoff-Khalsa, D. S. "Selective Unilateral Autonomic Activation: Implications for Psychiatry." *CNS Spectrums* 12, 8 (2007): 625–632.

Sivapriya, D. V., S. Malani, and S. Thirumeni. "Effect of Nadi Shodhana Pranayama on Respiratory Parameters in School Students." *Recent Research in Science and Technology* 2, no. 11 (2010): 32–39.

Telles, S., P. Raghuraj, M. Satyapriya, and H. R. Nagendra. "Immediate Effect of Three Yoga Breathing Techniques on Performance on a Letter-Cancellation Task." *Perceptual and Motor Skills* 104 (2007): 1289–1296.

Telles, S., A. Yadav, N. Kumar, S. Sharma, N. K. Visweshwarajah, and A. Balkrishna. "Blood Pressure and Purdue Pegboard Scores in Individuals with Hypertension after Alternate Nostril Breathing, Breath Awareness, and No Intervention." *Medical Science Monitor* 21, no. 19 (2013): 61–66.

Werntz, D. A., R. G. Bickford, F. E. Bloom, and D. S. Shannahoff-Khalsa. "Alternating Cerebral Hemispheric Activity and the Lateralization of Autonomic Nervous Function." *Human Neurobiology* 2 (1983): 39–43.

## CHAPTER 2

Jain, S., S. L. Shapiro, S. Swanick, S. C. Roesch, P. J. Mills, I. Bell, and G. E. Schwartz. "A Randomized Controlled Trial of Mindfulness Meditation versus Relaxation Training: Effects on Distress, Positive States of Mind, Rumination, and Distraction." *Annals of Behavioral Medicine* 33, no. 1 (2007): 11–21.

Levy, D. M., J. O. Wobbrock, A. W. Kaszniak, and M. Ostergren. "The Effects of Mindfulness Meditation Training on Multitasking in a High-Stress Information Environment." Paper presented at the Graphics Interface Conference, Toronto, Ontario, Canada, May 28–30, 2012.

## CHAPTER 3

Moyer, C. A., M. P. Donnelly, J. C. Anderson, K. C. Valek, S. J. Huckaby, R. L. Doty, A. S. Rehlinger, and B. L. Rice. "Frontal Electroencephalographic Asymmetry Associated with Positive Emotion Is Produced by Very Brief Meditation Training." *Psychological Science* 22, no. 10 (2011): 1277–1279.

Zeidan, F., N. S. Gordon, J. Merchant, and P. Goolkasian. "The Effects of Brief Mindfulness Meditation Training on Experimentally Induced Pain." *The Journal of Pain* 11, no. 3 (2010): 199–209.

## CHAPTER 5

Cahn, B. R., A. Delorme, and J. Polich. "Occipital Gamma Activation During Vipassana Meditation." *Cognitive Processing* 11, no. 1 (2010): 39–56.

Chiesa, A. "Zen Meditation: An Integration of Current Evidence." *Journal of Alternative and Complementary Medicine* 15, no. 5 (2009): 585–592.

Colzato, L. S., A. Ozturk, and B. Hommel. "Meditate to Create: The Impact of Focused-Attention and Open-Monitoring Training on Convergent and Divergent Thinking." *Frontiers in Psychology* 3 (2012): 116.

Grant, J. A. "Meditative Analgesia: The Current State of the Field." *Advances in Meditation Research: Neuroscience and Clinical Applications* 1307 (2014): 55–63.

Lippelt, D. P., B. Hommel, and L. S. Colzato. "Focused Attention, Open Monitoring and loving kindness Meditation: Effects on Attention, Conflict Monitoring and Creativity—A Review." *Frontiers in Psychology* 5 (2014): 1083.

Marzetti, L., C. Di Lanzo, F. Zappasodi, F. Chella, A. Raffone, and V. Pizella. "Magnetoencephalographic Alpha Band Connectivity Reveals Differential Default Mode Network Interactions During Focused Attention and Open Monitoring Meditation." *Frontiers in Human Neuroscience* 8 (2014): 832.

Perlman, D. M., T. V. Salomons, R. J. Davidson, and A. Lutz. "Differential Effects on Pain Intensity and Unpleasantness of Two Meditation Practices." *Emotion* 10, no. 1 (2010): 65–71.

Rubia, K. "The Neurobiology of Meditation and Its Clinical Effectiveness in Psychiatric Disorders." *Biological Psychology* 82, no. 1 (2009): 1–11.

Xu, J., A. Vik, I. R. Groote, J. Lagopoulos, A. Holen, O. Ellingsen, A. K. Haberg, and S. Davanger. "Nondirective Meditation Activated Default Mode Network Areas Associated with Memory Retrieval and Emotional Processing." *Frontiers in Human Neuroscience* 8 (2014): 86.

Zeidan, F., J. A. Grant, C. A. Brown, J. G. McHaffie, and R. C. Coghill. "Mindfulness Meditation-Related Pain Relief: Evidence for Unique Brain Mechanisms in the Regulation of Pain." *Neuroscience Letters* 520, no. 2 (2012): 165–173.

## CHAPTER 6

Hepworth, N. S. "A Mindful Eating Group as an Adjunct to Individual Treatment for Eating Disorders: A Pilot Study." *Eating Disorders: The Journal of Treatment and Prevention* 19, no. 1 (2010): 6–16.

Jordan, C. H., W. Wang, L. Donatoni, and B. P. Meier. "Mindful Eating: Trait and State Mindfulness Predicts Healthier Eating Behavior." *Personality and Individual Differences* 68 (2014): 107–111.

Kristeller, J. L., and R. Q. Wolever. "Mindfulness-Based Eating Awareness Training for Treating Binge Eating Disorder: The Conceptual Foundation." *Eating Disorders: The Journal of Treatment and Prevention* 19, no. 1 (2010): 49–61.

## CHAPTER 7

Condon, P., G. Desbordes, W. Miller, and D. DeSteno. "Meditation Increases Compassionate Responses to Suffering." *Psychological Science* 24, no. 10 (2013): 2125–2127.

Gard, T., B. K. Hölzel, A. T. Sack, H. Hempel, S. W. Lazar, D. Vaitl, and U. Ott. "Pain Attenuation through Mindfulness Is Associated with Decreased Cognitive Control and Increased Sensory Processing in the Brain." *Cerebral Cortex* 22, no. 11 (2012): 2692–2702.

Garland, E. L., S. A. Gaylord, O. Palsson, K. Faurot, J. Douglas Mann, and W. E. Whitehead. "Therapeutic Mechanisms of a Mindfulness-Based Treatment for IBS: Effects on Visceral Sensitivity, Catastrophizing, and Affective Processing of Pain Sensations." *Journal of Behavioral Medicine* 35, no. 6 (2012): 591–602.

Grant, J. A. "Meditative Analgesia: The Current State of the Field."*Advances in Meditation Research: Neuroscience and Clinical Applications* 1307 (2014): 55–63.

Mawani, A., S. Rashiq, M. J. Verrier, and B. D. Dick. "The Effect of Mindfulness Meditation on Pain and Spirituality in Patients with Chronic Non-Cancer Pain." *Journal of Pain Management* 7, no. 1 (2014): 75–82.

Morone, N. E., C. M. Greco, and D. K. Weiner. "Mindfulness Meditation for the Treatment of Chronic Low Back Pain in Older Adults: A Randomized Controlled Pilot Study." *Pain* 134 (2008): 310–319.

Perlman, D. M., T. V. Salomons, R. J. Davidson, and A. Lutz. "Differential Effects on Pain Intensity and Unpleasantness of Two Meditation Practices." *Emotion* 10, no. 1 (2010): 65–71.

Zeidan, F., J. A. Grant, C. A. Brown, J. G. McHaffie, and R. C. Coghill. "Mindfulness Meditation-Related Pain Relief: Evidence for Unique Brain Mechanisms in the Regulation of Pain." *Neuroscience Letters* 520, no. 2 (2012): 165–173.

Zeidan, F., K. T. Martucci, R. A. Kraft, N. K. Gordon, J. G. McHaffie, and R. C. Coghill. "Brain Mechanisms Supporting the Modulation of Pain by Mindfulness Meditation." *The Journal of Neuroscience* 31, no. 14 (2011): 5540–5548.

## CHAPTER 8

Borders, A., M. Earleywine, and A. Jajodia. "Could Mindfulness Decrease Anger, Hostility, and Aggression by Decreasing Rumination?" *Aggressive Behavior* 36, no. 1 (2010): 28–44.

Hölzel, B. K., J. Carmody, K. C. Evans, E. A. Hoge, J. A. Dusek, L. Morgan, R. K. Pitman, and S. W. Lazar. "Stress Reduction Correlates with Structural Changes in the Amygdala." *Social Cognitive and Affective Neuroscience* 5, no. 1 (2010): 11–17.

Hölzel, B. K., S. W. Lazar, T. Gard, Z. Schuman-Olivier, D. R. Vago, and U. Ott. "Does Mindfulness Meditation Work? Proposing Mechanisms of Action from a Conceptual and Neural Perspective." *Perspectives on Psychological Science* 6, no. 6 (2011): 537–539.

Jalaluddin, R., and C. Barks. *The Essential Rumi.* San Francisco: Harper Collins, 1996.

O'Connor, M., J. Piet, and E. Hougaard. "The Effects of Mindfulness-Based Cognitive Therapy on Depressive Symptoms in Elderly Bereaved People with Loss-Related Distress: A Controlled Pilot Study." *Mindfulness* 5, no. 4 (2014): 400–409.

Peters, J. R., L. M. Smart, T. A. Eisenlohr-Moul, P. J. Geiger, G. T. Smith, and R. A. Baer. "Anger Rumination as a Mediator of the Relationship between Mindfulness and Aggression: The Utility of a Multidimensional Mindfulness Model." *Journal of Clinical Psychology* 71, no. 9 (2015): 871–884.

Roberts, L. R., and S. B. Montgomery. "Mindfulness-Based Intervention for Perinatal Grief after Stillbirth in Rural India." *Issues in Mental Health Nursing* 36, no. 3 (2015): 222–230.

Tacon, A. M. "Mindfulness: Existential, Loss, and Grief Factors in Women with Breast Cancer." *Journal of Psychosocial Oncology* 29, no. 6 (2011): 643–656.

## CHAPTER 9

Cayoun, B. A. *Mindfulness-Integrated CBT: Principles and Practice.* Sussex, UK: Wiley-Blackwell, 2011.

Kuyken, W., R. Hayes, B. Barrett, et al. "Effectiveness and Cost-Effectiveness of Mindfulness-Based Cognitive Therapy Compared with Maintenance Antidepressant Treatment in the Prevention of Depressive Relapse or Recurrence (PREVENT): A Randomized Controlled Trial." *The Lancet* 386, no. 9988 (2015): 63–73.

Scheer, F. A. J. L., M. F. Hilton, C. S. Mantzoros, and S. A. Shea. "Adverse Metabolic and Cardiovascular Consequences of Circadian Misalignment." *Proceedings of the National Academy of Sciences of the United States of America* 106, no. 11 (2009): 4453–4458.

## CHAPTER 10

Desbordes, G., L. T. Negi, T. W. W. Pace, B. A. Wallace, C. J. Raison, and E. L. Schwartz. "Effects of Mindful-Attention and Compassion Meditation Training on Amygdala Response to Emotional Stimuli in an Ordinary, Non-Meditative State." *Frontiers in Human Neuroscience* 6, no. 292 (2012): 1–15.

Hutcherson, C. A., E. M. Seppala, and J. J. Gross. "The Neural Correlates of Social Connection." *Cognitive, Affective and Behavioural Neuroscience* 15, no. 1 (2015): 1–14.

Leary, M. R., E. B. Tate, C. E. Adams, A. B. Allen, and J. Hancock. "Self-Compassion and Reactions to Unpleasant Self-Relevant Events: The Implications of Treating Oneself Kindly." *Journal of Personality and Social Psychology* 92 (2007): 887–904.

Lee, T. M., M. K. Leung, W. K. Hou, J. C. Tang, J. Yin, K. F. So, C. F. Lee, and C. C. Chan. "Distinct Neural Activity Associated with Focused-Attention Meditation and loving kindness Meditation." *PLoS One* 7, no. 8 (2012): e40054.

Leung, M., C. C. H. Chan, J. Yin, C. Lee, K. So, and T. M. C. Lee. "Increased Gray Matter Volume in the Right Angular and Posterior Parahippocampal Gyri in loving kindness Meditators." *Social, Cognitive and Affective Neuroscience* 8, no. 1 (2013): 34–39.

Lutz, A., J. Brefczynski-Lewis, T. Johnstone, and R. J. Davidson. "Regulation of the Neural Circuitry of Emotion by Compassion Meditation: Effects of Meditative Expertise." *PLOS One* 3, no. 3 (2008): e1897.

Lutz, A., L. L. Greischar, D. M. Perlman, and R. J. Davidson. "BOLD Signal in Insula Is Differentially Related to Cardiac Function During Compassion Meditation in Experts vs Novices." *NeuroImage* 47 (2009): 1038–1046.

McKnight, D. E. "Tonglen Meditation's Effect on Compassion in Novice Meditators." Unpublished Ph.D. diss., University of the West, 2014. http://gradworks.umi.com/36/31/3631403.html.

Neff, K. D., and C. K. Germer. "A Pilot Study and Randomized Controlled Trial of the Mindful Self-Compassion Program." *Journal of Clinical Psychology* 69, no. 1 (2012): 28–44.

Neff, K. D., Y. Hseih, and K. Dejitthirat. "Self-Compassion, Achievement Goals, and Coping with Academic Failure." *Self and Identity* 4 (2005): 263–287.

Rockliff, H., P. Gilbert, K. McEwan, S. Lightman, and D. Glover. "A Pilot Exploration of Heart Rate Variability and Salivary Cortisol Responses to Compassion-Focused Imagery." *Clinical Neuropsychiatry* 5 (2008): 132–139.

Weng, H. Y., A. S. Fox, A. J. Shackman, D. E. Stodola, J. Z. K. Caldwell, M. C. Olson, G. M. Rogers, and R. J. Davidson. "Compassion Training Alters Altruism and Neural Responses to Suffering." *Psychological Science* 24, no. 7 (2013): 1171–1180.

## SUMMARY

Desikachar, T. K. V. *The Heart of Yoga*. Rochester, VT: Inner Traditions International, 1995.

## Q&A

Cayoun, B. A. Mindfulness-Integrated CBT: Principles and Practice. Sussex, UK: Wiley-Blackwell, 2011.

# Index